MIND YOUR BODY

FEB. 2008

CATALINA:

MIND YOUR BODY!

MIND YOUR BODY

PILATES FOR THE SEATED PROFESSIONAL

BY JULI KAGAN

MINDBODY
PUBLISHING

For further information, please contact:

MindBody Publishing
www.MindYourBodyBook.com

Book design by:

VMC Art & Design LLC
P.O. Box 153
Allendale, NJ 07401
info@vmc-artdesign.com
www.vmc-artdesign.com

Photography by Gonzalo Villota
www.villota.com
info@villota.com

Printed in the United States of America

Mind Your Body—Pilates for the Seated Professional
Juli Kagan

1. Title 2. Author 3. Health and Fitness

Library of Congress Control Number: 2006928969

ISBN 10 : 0-9787145-0-4
ISBN 13: 978-0-9787145-0-5

MEDICAL DISCLAIMER:

If during any of the exercises you experience pain or unusual discomfort you should cease the exercise immediately, as Pilates should not hurt. Pilates' exercises will push you beyond yourself; however, this is achieved with respect to all the Pilates principles throughout the exercises. You should seek the guidance from your personal health professional before beginning any exercise regime.

DEDICATION

To Zachary: my teacher and true inspiration—in every sense of the word.
Thank you for being you!
To David: my rock. I am so grateful for your unconditional love
and the freedom you give me to be me.

ACKNOWLEDGEMENTS

Writing a book is not a simple task and is the accrual of many years of learning—my favorite endeavor. It also takes many talented people to pull it together.

The following people have helped make my goals a reality and for that I am extremely appreciative:

To my Mom and Dad: for always believing in me.

To my entire immediate family: for your constant love and endless understanding.

To my extended "family" of professors and students at Nova Dental School and Broward Community College, as well as Royal Palm Yacht and Country Club: you are my true motivation and the reason I know I am supposed to be a teacher here on this earth.

To my dear friends and colleagues: you are the scaffolding of my life. What would I do without you?

To photographer extraordinaire Gonzalo Villota: your methodical work is brilliant. So are you. Thank you!

To my phenomenal editors, Ali Kaufman & Alison Moore: you made my book come to life! I am forever indebted to each of you.

To graphic designer Victoria Colotta: you saved my book and continued to lead the way despite many challenges. My deepest gratitude to you!

To Monica, Dr. Rich, and Alison: you were the chosen ones because you "get it!" Thanks!

To all of my readers: knowledge is power—harness it, make better choices, but mostly, move!

CONTENTS

INTRODUCTION

I have dedicated my life melding physical and mental fitness. With three certifications in Pilates, two degrees in dental hygiene, and a Masters Degree in Educational Psychology, my unique perspective is driven by the culmination of more than 25 years spent in both the fitness and dental fields. I teach my students and address my readers from a unique knowledge base, which I apply from a holistic perspective: every aspect of our physical and mental health is interwoven.

My knowledge and experience is the compilation of a lifetime of physical activity and applied learning, as well as on-the-job observing and ergonomics training. The awareness I have gained from my own fitness background and from helping my clients reset their own posture, reclaim their breathing power, and redesign their work-a-day habits has led to the publication of this book—the first to outline a Pilates-based workout targeting seated professionals.

Originally this book was meant to be a manual for dental professionals. However, while writing, it became clear that all professionals are at similar risk of occupational injury resulting from situational and postural hazards in todays work environment. One would expect health risks on the job if you report to work every day in a coal mine, but not working behind a desk; yet the risks are everywhere. The problem is, today's busy professionals don't have time to stop, pay attention, and prevent injury. Whatever your work environment, one thing is clear: you are at risk for musculo-skeletal injury in every physical position.

As a professor of ergonomics and instrumentation at Nova Dental School in Fort Lauderdale, Florida, I teach students to understand and address the physical strain they will face in their professional lives by introducing them to the positive effects mindful movement can have on their job satisfaction, career development, patient care, and lifelong health.

Every position we move in and out of is the result of both a physical and mental choice. In 1999, I made a connection that had previously eluded me throughout all of the physical activities I had participated in until then. I took a Pilates class. I had been a gymnast, a runner, an aerobics enthusiast and instructor, and even a martial artist and long distance bicycler. However, it wasn't until my first Pilates lesson that I finally understood the importance of making a body-mind-spirit connection in my exercise program.

Pilates offered me what the other regimes didn't: a fitness program that combined the physical aspects of exercising, without all of the sweat, repetition, and boredom of my previous activities. Plus, Pilates offered me another bonus, an introduction to the importance of mental clarity and precise posture.

I wish for all of my readers, whatever your profession, a lifetime of mindful movements, full breaths, and positive intentions.

MIND YOUR BODY

PILATES FOR THE SEATED PROFESSIONAL

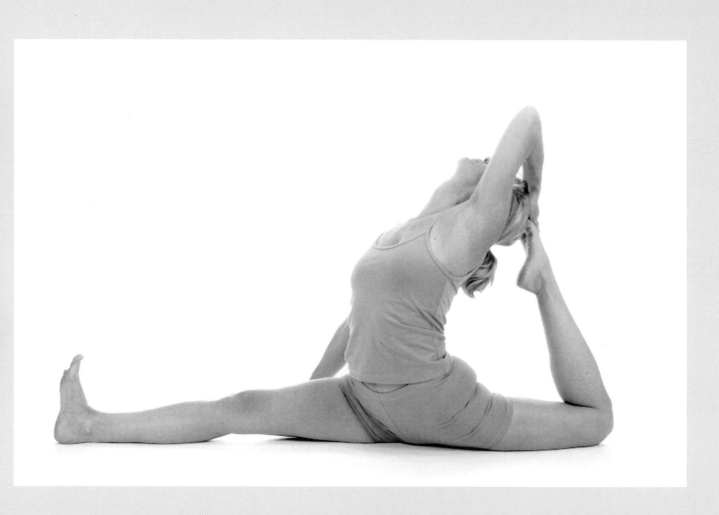

PART 1:

A WORKFORCE IN CRISIS

The seated professional is in a postural crisis. On a monthly basis, popular magazine and professional journal articles focus on the biomechanical problems that cause the aches, pains, and disorders, that can make life miserable for people who are seated. While no one is immune, those in the work environment are especially susceptible to these types of complaints and disorders. It affects the receptionist awkwardly cradling the phone in between the ear and shoulder, the person working on a computer who often slouches to type and gets tired viewing the monitor, or the professional who is often in the same forced position for long periods of time. Now add emotional and mental stress and the result is often debilitating.

Unfortunately, knowing better doesn't always translate into doing better. You know you shouldn't cramp your neck or shoulder to hold the phone, you know you shouldn't lean over the keyboard or monitor, but you do these things anyway. You also know you can stretch to relieve tight muscles; unfortunately you just don't.

Despite the availability of ergonomic chairs and work spaces, and the plethora of information on preventive back care, the fact remains that you still suffer aching joints and muscles due to awkward and precarious positions.

HOW IS THE SEATED PROFESSIONAL REALLY DOING?

Very controlled, forced and awkward positions are often overwhelming to the body's structural system due to the repetitive nature of tasks and time spent performing them. Modern conveniences such as the computer, while improving job performance and productivity, keep us in positions which are not suited to our anatomy.

The U.S. Department of Labor's Bureau of Labor Statistics reported approximately 706,000 cases of overexertion or repetitive motion injuries in the most recent published reports. Of these, 367,000, or approximately one half, affected the back. Almost 100,000 of the injuries were due to repetitive motion, including typing or key entry, repetitive use of tools, and repetitive placing, grasping, or moving objects that affected the wrist, shoulder and back.

A substantial body of credible epidemiological research provides strong evidence of an association between musculoskeletal disorders and specific physical exposures, especially when they are intense, prolonged, and when workers are exposed to several risk factors simultaneously.

When we designed more automated workplaces, we aimed to take the pressure off our body. For example, in the 1960's, dentists were trained to sit, rather than stand when practicing, to alleviate lower extremity pain. However, sitting presented a whole new set of problems. When seated, the pressure on soft tissue structures of the lower lumbar spine and the discs between the spinal vertebrae is increased. In addition, one must add harmful spinal twisting and rotation, forward and side bending, and awkward body alignment throughout the day.

These **strained postures can result in muscle stiffness and tightening, which often leads to surging pain, causing further immobility.** The resultant absence of motion causes more stiffening, which leads to further tightening and more severe muscular back pain. The cycle is vicious and debilitating.

WHAT'S YOUR POSTURE ID?

If proper posture is the goal, what shape are you in now? Take a few moments to assess your natural seated position. Make sure to consider all of the places that you sit: your desk, the conference room, your car, your kitchen table, your couch…If you really want to get your facts, have a family member, friend or co-worker photograph you in the seated position when you least expect it.

When you have assessed your posture mentally or even made up a list and possibly taken your photos, use these Posture ID descriptions to see how you shape up.

THE SHIFTER

You can't sit in the middle of the chair because you are always sitting on one side or the other, towards the edge, or in motion from one position to another. No position is ever neutral or comfortable.

THE LEANER

You never sit completely straight; your head, neck, and spine appear to be almost floppy and fluid, while the bottom half of the body stays stable.

THE ROUNDER

You "hunchback," bent at mid-chest level. The spine appears to be shaped like the letter 'C'.

THE SLOUCHER

You just can't "Sit up straight!" You have a tendency to bend at the lower back from a lazy lumbar.

THE NECK-CRANER

You stretch your neck out of alignment constantly, for example, by holding a phone to your ear.

THE STRAIGHT SITTER

You sit balanced in the seat, spine erect; head held high, and hips and shoulders in neutral. Most often you have a smile and positive outlook!

As you continue through this book and experiment with The Exercises, see if your Posture ID changes.

A PAIN IN THE NECK

Seated professionals are particularly prone to tension in the neck, due to dysfunction or over function of the muscles of the shoulders, neck and back. Spinal trouble often results as a cascading sequela to these overtaxed muscles. As you can surmise, spinal instability and spinal pain go hand-in-hand.

If your lower back or upper shoulders are often strained **and fatigued, it is almost** *certain that your posture, muscles, ligaments, joints, tendons and bones are not balanced.* Both your alignment and strength will improve when you can decrease the strain on the musculoskeletal system. However, reducing the strain requires changing your most basic postural habits.

There are many other bad habits the seated professional must consider regarding back and shoulder pain. Firstly, you routinely shift between awkward positions, especially after sitting for long periods of time; second, you are required to do repetitive motions throughout the day; and third, you are often under inordinate stress, causing you to unconsciously tighten your muscles, which exacerbates an already compromised musculoskeletal system.

It is astounding that so little preventive care and attention is given to the seated professional regarding back care, upper body exercises and what can be done proactively to prevent postural and bodily harm. Without preventative measures the consequences can be serious. The resulting dysfunctional spine and weak upper body invariably leads to pain, missed work, early forced retirement, and medical interventions- to say nothing of the economic hardship that follows. It is most regrettable that a well-organized professional who excels at time management and the fulfillment of established objectives on the job would be inattentive to his or her own physical health and well-being.

One thing is certain, the need for spinal alignment and realignment is constant. *When you sit or stand with your spine warped, your body will compensate and create sophisticated ways of counter acting and counter balancing muscle discrepancies.* Unfortunately, this effort will often cause more unnatural and less desirable movements, which can lead to future pain and injury. The cycle must be intercepted. Knowledge and mind-body awareness is a beginning in the right direction. Exercising, stretching and Pilates will break the cycle.

Pilates and the stretching exercises in this book, when practiced consistently, are the keys to maintaining both physical and mental health for the seated professional. Indeed exercise and the resulting focus on posture can change your life!

MY STORY

For as long as I can remember, being involved in some form of physical activity has been important. As a youngster and accomplished gymnast, working out four hours a day after school was my routine. The control, balance and coordination gained was remarkable. As a teen, running kept my weight in check. During college, I had heard that weight gain was more probable than at any other time in life, so I was bound and determined to avoid that phenomenon. I ran along the Charles River, at least 5 times a week, while attending Forsyth School for Dental Hygiene in Boston. Becoming keenly interested in nutrition, I took elective courses that would help me to maintain a healthy body. As a young adult I taught aerobics and went to the gym and took part in body conditioning programs, step classes, etc. Later, I took up weight training and participated in a triathlon. Exercise and being active were cornerstones of my life and certainly influenced some of the qualities I posses now including: discipline, an awareness of my own body, and vitality.

At the age of 30 I became pregnant. Within six weeks after the birth of my son, my weight and physique were back to normal, although my breasts were a bit larger from nursing! The rapid physical changes were likely attributed to everything I had learned and applied before the nine months of gestation-exercising regularly, eating sensibly, and mostly, listening to my body. Later in life, I became a brown belt in Kenpo Style Martial Arts and then started biking and spinning. I even did a 250-mile AIDS ride!

In 1999, I found myself at a Pilates class. *Little did I know that of all the exercise regimens I had been involved with, throughout my entire life, that Pilates would reverberate and resonate so strongly with my body, mind, and spirit!* I had finally found something that brought together the physical aspects of exercising with the mental health benefits of focus. The repetition and boredom, which were increasingly plaguing me under my previous exercise regimens, were gone. I was hooked and working from my core, both figuratively and literally!

THE PILATES CHRONOLOGY

The Pilates Method of exercise and wellness was the brainchild of Joseph Pilates. Not blessed with good health as a child, Joseph sought to reverse his suffering as an adult. Growing up, his body was wrought with frailties, including asthma, rheumatic fever, and rickets. The Pilates Method grew from his obsession with overcoming these maladies and restoring his physical well being. In devising his method of breathing, body awareness, and movement, he merged Western forms of physical studies with Eastern forms of exercise. What resulted has changed the course of many lives since Joseph Pilates first changed his own.

While at a British internment camp, in 1918, Pilates' compatriots followed his exercise routine in the hopes of warding off the influenza epidemic of the time. When none of his trainees' died from the flu, the Pilates method began to gain popularity through its credibility as a preventive measure against sickness.

Perhaps most interesting was the equipment Pilates fashioned together to help bedridden patients regain their health. He created unique apparatus that employed bedsprings to provide resistance, while pulleys made from leather and rope guided the patients' movements and helped lengthen their extremities. His most popular piece of equipment, known as a reformer, has changed little and is still considered a brilliantly engineered piece of exercise equipment.

The first Pilates Studio opened when he immigrated to the United States in 1926, and the Pilates Method has changed little since then. From the days when dancers and performers like Balanchine were his students, to today, successful professionals credit Pilates with their heightened mind/body balance.

A NEW WAY TO WORK OUT

Pilates will change the way you think about exercise. It will also change the way you generally function and move throughout your day. **A Pilates workout is unlike any other exercise program you have ever done. First-timers often finish a session saying, "I have never felt like this before!"**

Pilates takes less than an hour per exercise period and all you really need is three times a week. **More is not always better. Effectiveness and efficiency go hand-in-hand.** It is Pilates himself who said, "Man should bear in mind and ponder over the Greek admonition-not too much, not too little." We've heard it enough-everything in moderation! Patience and practice are keys-just like anything worth their potential.

As you do Pilates and other stretching exercises, you will immediately feel better. I have heard this from students/practitioners over and over again. **As the Chinese say, you are as old as your spine is flexible. So, how old is your spine?** I am hopeful that if you choose to consistently exercise you will feel younger and more supple everyday.

Students love Pilates because it's not boring. That is because the exercises, selected by the instructor from a large variety, are performed in a specific order to achieve targeted results. There are only a small number of repetitions for each exercise, making each workout both interesting and efficient. In addition, when you have performed the exercises methodically and precisely you are totally challenged without creating what Pilates called "muscular-fatigue poison," otherwise known as lactic acid build-up.

Unlike most other forms of exercise, you end each Pilates session with a feeling of invigoration and contentment, instead of relief that the session is over. This is due to the fact that Pilates encourages an attention to breathing, with an emphasis on full inhalations and even more complete exhalations. It is the antithesis of running on a treadmill utilizing incomplete cycles of shallow breathing or panting. This focus on oxygen usage ensures that exhaustion does not take hold.

> ### TRY THIS!
>
> On your next breathing break, take a few deep breaths while imagining that helium is lifting your head off of your shoulders. At the same time, as you feel your head rise from the crown, tighten your abdominals and elongate the spine from the base of your tailbone to the top of your head.
>
> *A few breathing breaks a day*
> *helps keep the tension away!*

TAKE TWO BREATHS AND CALL ME IN THE MORNING

The breath is an unrivaled elixir, and Joseph Pilates encouraged a consistent dosage of inhalations and exhalations. Medical professionals already understand the link between breathing and calming. When we administer local anesthesia to a nervous patient, we say, "take a deep breath" before inserting the needle. We know that a deep breath is an antidote to physical stress. After a long, hard day, don't you often take a deep inhale and an even deeper exhale to relieve nervous tension? **Our breath carries many curative and restorative properties.** Breath work is vital to a healthy life and imperative to the Pilates Method.

WANT A SMARTER BODY?

The more you do Pilates, the more you learn about the function of your own body.

The key to a smarter body is making smarter movements and holding smarter postures. Conscious movements sharpen your defenses against musculoskeletal damage. *Pilates mobilizes and releases stiff muscles so they become lithe and more flexible.* The exercises are both supportive and gentle. *They target the back, core, shoulder girdle and upper trunk-all areas seated professionals risk injuring.* After only a few short sessions, you will notice yourself making intuitive minor adjustments to your positioning. You will sit, stand, and move with a heightened awareness of your physical stability and composure.

Nothing is more important than spinal health; ask anyone with a back issue! When the back is strong and the core muscles work in unison with the back, posture is almost guaranteed to be intact.

SEATED ASSESSMENT

Use this checklist to make sure you are sitting correctly as you work:

- Keep your feet flat.
- Keep your ankles and knees at 90-degree angles.
- Sit in your chair with your hips open to about 130 degree angle between your abdomen and thighs.
- Sit IN the chair, and not OFF of the chair.
- Pull your navel in gently.
- Your back should be erect and gently lifted.
- Let your shoulder blades gently glide down your upper back.
- Let your neck release into a neutral position.
- Keep your shoulders balanced and square over your center.
- Balance your hips.
- Your arms should be parallel to, or higher than, the floor (between 80-110 degrees, and slightly away from your body).
- Maintain rhythmic breathing, taking full inhalations and exhalations.

WHY PILATES IS SO GOOD FOR YOU!

While Pilates is different from other forms of exercise, it also compliments them. It is different because the focus is primarily based around core strengthening-a MUST for the seated professional. You train the abdominal muscles to control all other movements. As a matter of fact, this is how most of the Pilates exercises are executed. *The core is primary and the extremities are secondary.* Most other forms of strength and flexibility training focus primarily on the specific limb or extremity itself (i.e. arm curls to strengthen the biceps.) **Pilates strengthens the muscle at its stretched and lengthened position, allowing the muscle to become longer and leaner without building bulk.**

PILATES SPECIFICALLY HELPS THE
SEATED PROFESSIONAL:

- Develop core abdominal strength, which is especially imperative for a person who sits in a chair most of the day.
- Develop the deepest muscles of the body to build strength and control.
- Improve mind/body awareness.
- Exercise muscles without causing pain.
- Move and exercise in a way that will not risk tearing muscles or jamming joints.
- Learn to feel a freedom of movement instead of straining muscles while functioning.
- Enhance muscle control without causing tension.
- Relieve any current pain, stiffness and/or tension and help prevent maladies.
- Reduce stress and fatigue.
- Feel invigorated and revitalized.
- Develop a longer, leaner body by lengthening and strengthening the muscles without creating bulk.

I like Pilates better than any other discipline because **Pilates is for the thinker; one truly uses the mind, directing the body to do the work.** Making this mental and physical connection is exceptionally powerful and empowering! You will both crave and channel this level of engagement- and not just in your workouts. Your mindfulness in living your life will go up and your level of stress will go down. How can you not love that?

KEEP MOVING

One last thought before you read on: Pilates is not an overnight cure. It is, however, your best prevention against spinal deterioration. Reading this book is the first step toward pain-free workdays, but you also have to do the work. Do every exercise with awareness and intention. Engage your mind AND body in your work. Move consciously, breathe deeply, and you will end up sitting and standing erect with your shoulders back, neck long, and spine tall.

AS PROFESSIONALS WITH BUSY LIVES, WE DON'T HAVE TIME FOR EVERY-THING WE WOULD LIKE TO BE ABLE TO DO. WE MUST CHOOSE WHICH THINGS ARE THE MOST IMPORTANT TO US AND WILL HAVE THE GREAT-EST POSITIVE INFLUENCE ON OUR LIVES FOR THE TIME AND EFFORT EX-PENDED. I PROMISE YOU, PILATES IS WELL WORTH THIS INVESTMENT.

"Contrology" (also known as "Pilates"), is designed to give you suppleness, natural grace and skill that will be unmistakably reflected in the way you walk, in the way you play, and in the way you work. You will develop muscular power with corresponding endurance, an ability to perform arduous duties, to play strenuous games, to walk, run, or travel for long distances without undue body fatigue or mental strain."

—Joseph Pilates

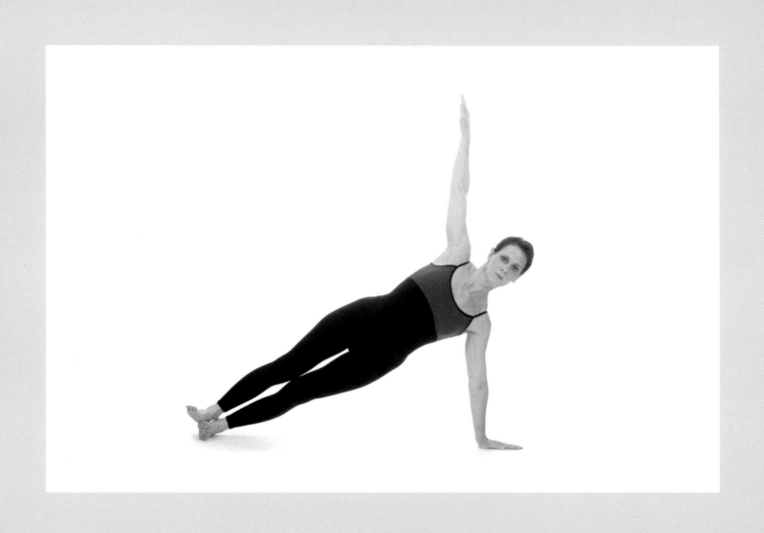

PART 2:

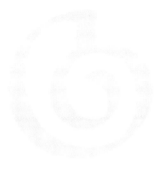

STRAIGHTEN UP

YOUR POSTURE SAYS
A LOT ABOUT YOU

When you stand, what are you projecting to the world? Are your shoulders broad and confident or round and guarded? Is your spine straight, curved, or hunched? You may find that you aren't very happy with the answer. Many seated professionals, especially those who lean over a computer are notoriously known to exhibit an awkward arched posture.

THERE'S NO SUCH THING AS
A SECOND IMPRESSION

The impression you make in the workplace establishes the tone for all of your professional relationships and accomplishments. A firm handshake, genuine smile and continuous eye contact are often indicators of a vital first impression. Remember, proper posture inspires confidence and trust with your colleagues, clients and customers, and is a strong suggestion of your character and disposition.

Impressive posture goes a long way. For example, if you were to choose a new business consultant and given two to choose from, both equally credentialed, but one's posture was straight and the other slouched, who do you think you would choose? Subliminally, most would choose the professional with the straighter posture. Where do you stand?

LISTEN UP!

One of the greatest problems today's professionals face is that when we get a slight twinge of pain or discomfort while working, we ignore it. This leads us to work through the discomfort until it just becomes routine to do so. We have, until now, assumed that the pain was just the cost of doing business. However, the pain actually costs us more in the end. After all, when the body finally does exhibit pain, it's long after the structural damage to tissues, muscles, tendons, ligaments, and joints has begun. **Your body is trying to tell you something when it is in pain- pay attention.**

A POSTURE CHECK-UP

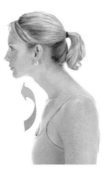

It's time to see where, or rather how, you stand. If you can have someone take a photo of you standing, while you least suspect it, that would be ideal. Otherwise, a quick mental snapshot in a mirror can suffice.

Most people exhibit one or more of the following: the chin is down or protruding forward, the shoulders are rolled forward, the abdomen is loose and the belly is sticking out, and/or the low back is curved excessively.

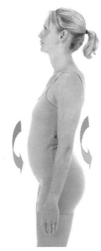

To realign your body, stand and try the following:

1. Elongate your tailbone towards the floor without jutting your pelvis under forcefully.

2. Align your pelvis so that the hipbones are parallel to the pubic bone.

3. Engage your abdominals by bringing your navel towards your spine. Imagine pulling on a tight pair of jeans; now release the effort 10%.

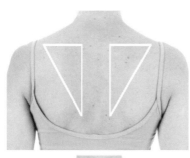

4. Next, roll your shoulder blades along your back ribs, as if the base of the shoulder blade was reaching toward imaginary back pants pockets. Don't over contract the muscles between the shoulder blades in order to accomplish this. Simply melt and draw your shoulder blades down your back. This indirectly opens the collar bones, which opens the chest, which allows for more effective and efficient breathing!

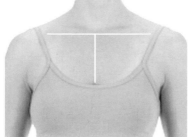

5. Look for parallelism of the collarbones to the floor. Determine if the chest plate is perpendicular to the collarbones. Stand proud, with your chest lifted and all tension released.

Stand relaxed, arms by your side and draw a line, connecting imaginary dots at the ankle, hip joint, corner of the shoulder and lobe of your ear. When these landmarks line-up, your posture is ideal. If you are one of the many for whom these dots don't connect, becoming aware of your postural tendencies is the first step towards improving your alignment-and your health.

"Nature has endowed human beings with a backbone, but few realize the state of perfection in which the "ridgepole" of the human "house" may properly grow into a normal, straight form as nature intended. Even fewer understand the mechanism of the spine and the proper methods of training this foundation of the body so that its movements will be under their absolute control at all times. The human spine has been sadly neglected for many, many generations."

— Joseph Pilates

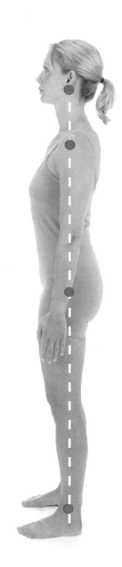

THE SPINE SPEAKS

Your spinal cord transmits communications between your brain and body. When your spine is aligned, these messages flow freely. However, when your "body is in knots," the brain's messages are blocked by individual vertebra that are not in communication with the motherboard.

How does the spine communicate? The spine is engineered to communicate through motion. The suppleness of the spine depends on the lubricating properties of the discs between each vertebra, which cushions the movements. **Spinal alignment can be likened to the cascading of a waterfall or to a row of dominoes falling down one by one. Each vertebra falls into its rightful place, as if they were a stack of blocks, built edge-to-edge and corner-to-corner.**

When all the parts of the spine are aligned and functionally interrelated, the spine performs at its highest capacity. A spine performing below capacity would induce symptoms like nerve impingement, compressed disks, weakened bones, and other postural-related ailments. Often, the physical weakness ultimately becomes emotional stress. Pilates is one of the most effective ways to treat both the emotional and physical burdens stress places on the body, especially the spine.

WHAT JOE REALLY THOUGHT

When Pilates trained his ballerinas or boxers who had foot or hand problems, he always started with the core and stabilizing muscles of the back. **Pilates did not believe in treating the specific extremity or body part. Rather, he focused on creating a strong center and above all, was very attentive to breath.**

Pilates believed oxygen was a large part of the healing process. His focus was on movement, mind and breath, and developed a proven method to circulate the blood, which supplied oxygen to ailing body parts.

With our current knowledge about the role that the mind and breath play regarding healing, there is no wonder that Pilates was on target and way ahead of his time. The bottom line is that his clients, often bedridden and disadvantaged, got better when he trained them.

"Physical fitness is the first requisite of happiness. It is the attainment and maintenance of a uniformly developed body as well as a sound mind, fully capable of naturally, easily, and satisfactorily performing our many and varied daily tasks with spontaneous zest and pleasure."

— Joseph Pilates

MOVE MORE, WORK BETTER

It's actually quite important to move more in order to work better. In order to boost your energy level and your productivity, look for ways to change your position throughout your workday. Here are a few tips to integrate movement into your workday:

- When you can, take a phone call standing up. Moving from a sitting to a standing position gives the pelvic girdle a rest and at the same time allows the joint to become more neutral and natural in its alignment.

- Of course, if you must sit, sit correctly. Your pelvis is shaped like a large salad bowl, with a base smaller than its rim. When most of us sit, however, we often sit on the side of the base, rather than its center. Try to be mindful of centering your pelvis as you sit.

- Don't forget to breathe! Taking deep breaths is the best way to keep your energy up and your stress level down.

PILATES ANATOMY 101

Sometimes you will hear the term "core" used to represent muscles of the abdominal area. The main muscles responsible for good posture are the core stabilizing muscles: the abdominals, back, buttocks and pelvic floor muscles. Envision a pair of bicycle shorts to help clarify the muscles of and around the core. Joseph Pilates coined this grouping of muscles the "powerhouse" and it truly is where one derives power and where overall body strength is housed. Importantly, **the stronger the interior muscles, the better the backbone will be supported. A stable spine and back is one that is strong as well as flexible.**

The nucleus of our "functional anatomy" is the powerhouse. It is this vital area, our true center, which supplies our most vital energy and strength. In mainstream workouts, we are conditioned to believe that working our extremities, or arms and legs, is the key to a complete workout. However, **as Pilates proves, function and performance is stored and cultivated in our core.**

Pilates works from the inside of the body first, so the weaker muscles of the core, or trunk area, and back become stronger. When alignment is achieved, and the spine is stable and upright, the spinal ligaments, skeletal bones, muscular and central nervous systems are all in accord.

TRY THIS!

Remember this checklist and adjust your standing posture when necessary:

⑥ The neck is long

⑥ The shoulders are down

⑥ The waist is lengthened on the sides and pulled in and up at the center

⑥ The spine is sturdy and straight

⑥ The legs are at their greatest length

⑥ The feet are firmly placed on the ground

With this alignment you will feel stretched and strong. Just what Pilates would have intended!

MUSCLES AND MORE

Learning the names of the muscles below is not for testing purposes. The reason for describing them is simply to help you understand what you may be specifically feeling as you begin the work.

The primary muscles of the powerhouse are the "abdominals" including: the rectus abdominis, external & internal obliques, and transversus abdominis, listed from most outside to most interior.

The **rectus abdominis** is what is popularly known as the "six pack." This long muscle runs from the top of the pubic bone to the chest plate and is responsible for forward bending at the waist.

The **external and internal obliques** run downward and upward and literally hug your waist. They function to compress the abdomen and move the torso in order to twist and turn.

The **transversus abdominis** is the deepest muscle, and wraps around from the back to the front, like a girdle across the abdomen. It applies pressure to the tummy and holds the organs in place. When

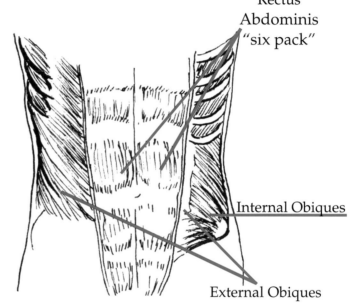

Rectus Abdominis "six pack"

Internal Obiques

External Obiques

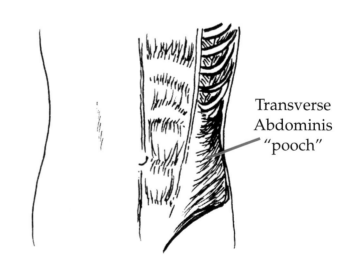

Transverse Abdominis "pooch"

you sneeze or cough, this muscle is strongly contracted. When it is weak in women, it is often exhibited as a "pooch."

The abdominal muscles collectively function to move and stabilize the spine and trunk, and without a doubt, are the most important muscles influencing posture.

The most important muscles, after the abdominals, when working in a seated position are the spine extensors, which include three pairs of muscles known collectively as erector spinae. They run from the hip to the neck on both sides of the spinal column and branch off to the ribs and spine. Obviously, their function is to keep the spine erect and the body upright. When only one side contracts, the spine bends to that side only.

Two other smaller but important muscles of the back include: the lumbar multifidus and quadratus lumborum. The lumbar multifidus allows the vertebra to attach to each other and the spinal column in a specialized arrangement, holding together each vertebra on their wings. Although this muscle has

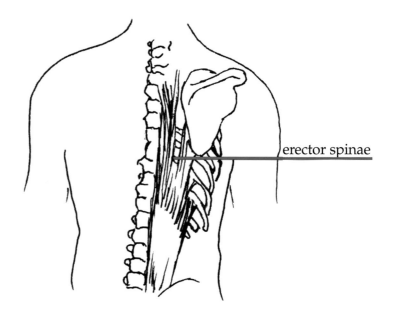

erector spinae

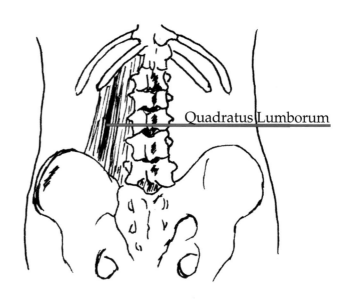

Quadratus Lumborum

21

insignificant large motor function, it functions primarily to maintain the spinal column.

The quadratus lumborum is a deep interior waist muscle. It assists in extending and lifting the spine, but it functions primarily in bending the torso sideways. This muscle often gets taxed when you lean over your chair, reaching for something, and balance to "hang on" to a position!

In general, the transversus abdominis and lumbar multifidus muscles are important in seated work as they maintain spinal stability and optimal alignment.

Lastly, the lumbar spine can also become compromised when the hamstrings (muscles behind the thighs) and the gluteal (butt) muscles are inflexible. Both help in daily locomotion. We sit on these muscles all day!

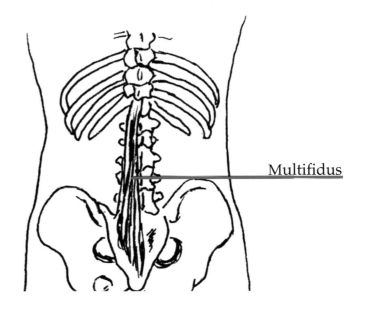

Multifidus

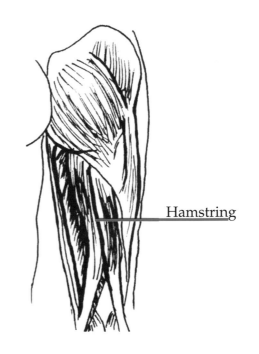

Hamstring

LET'S GET STARTED

So far, you have read about the fundamentals of Pilates for the seated professional. Now it's time to put words into action. A final note, however. **Pilates is complimentary to other exercise programs as it enhances, improves and supports all other exercise modalities.** I recommend you still run, swim, bike or work on an elliptical machine for cardiovascular health and endurance. Please continue to play tennis, golf, basketball or other sports to practice balance and coordination. Lift weights for muscle and bone strength. These all work beautifully in conjunction with Pilates which will actually enhance and improve your physical condition for each discipline.

Lastly, Pilates works because it makes you more aware of your body. You become your own body expert, intricately attentive to its strengths and weaknesses. Pilates will help you find balance within yourself and within your physical environment. And yes, you will become much more aware of your posture, spinal alignment, and sense of being after only a few sessions. Let's get started! I can't wait to hear your positive stories.

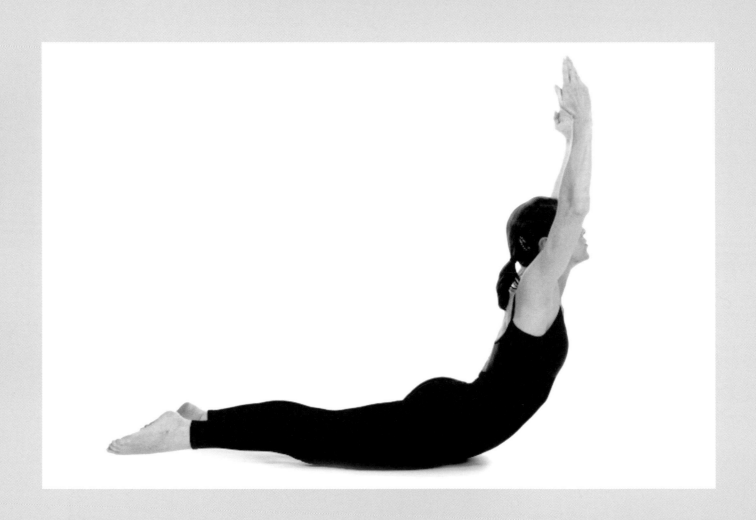

PART 3:

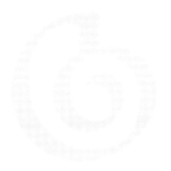

S.O.S.! SAVE OUR SPINES!

RESPECT YOUR SPINE

With a clear understanding of anatomy, you can now see that the spine is the center of your alignment, literally and figuratively. Think of the spine as a vertical pole with two horizontal rods emanating from it. These rods represent the shoulders and hips with the arms and legs hanging from them. The center pole is foundational. It supports everything! It balances everything and creates our portability, poise, and pride.

Have you ever seen a person whose back is round and bent forward (called kyphosis)? Think of an older woman suffering with osteoporosis. In more severe cases this is known as a Dowager's hunchback. Seated professionals, especially those hunched over a computer are notoriously known to exhibit this posture. (See *"What's You Posture ID—The Rounder"* on page 3.) Remember that the spine is virtuous—it should be treated with the respect and reverence it is due.

PRINCIPLES AT WORK

Before you begin the exercise program and in order to serve your spine effectively and efficiently, it is helpful to understand a set of principles Pilates believed would enhance the quality of each movement. These principles allow you to practice in a balanced, sensible way with an awareness of confidence, grace, and style. As you will come to find, **quality of movement is much more important than quantity of repetitions.**

Individually, the principles seem quite attainable. It is when you can master them in unison, and cooperatively, that enormous benefit and effect will come about. It is akin to the ease with which an ice dancer lifts his partner in the air. It looks so effortless, yet much training went into all the parts.

These principles can enhance your performance in just about any activity. However, in the workplace, when practiced regularly, these principles will ensure both physical and mental victory.

THE PILATES PRINCIPLES INCLUDE:

- Breathing
- Concentration
- Centering
- Control
- Flow
- Flexibility
- Precision
- Routine

BREATHING

Joseph Pilates taught his students, "Above all, learn to breathe correctly." As we have established, **the breath is the momentum that sends the blood flowing through your body.** A strong, deep breath is paramount to spinal health. A shallow breath will contribute to stagnation, lethargy, and mental misfiring.

"Completely inhaling and exhaling supplies the bloodstream with vital necessary life-giving oxygen from the tips of your fingers to the toes. Breathing is the first act of life, and the last. Our very life depends on it. Correct breathing will result in the bloodstream receiving its full quota of oxygen and thus ward off undue fatigue."

—Joseph Pilates

Learning how to contract the abdominal muscles while simultaneously breathing is foundational in every Pilates exercise. Breathing into the bottom of your lungs and taking full breaths, both inhaling and fully exhaling is essential and challenging. It is the antithesis of a "muscle jock," who holds his breath while lifting a heavy weight thereby creating incredible intrathoracic pressure. In Pilates, the inhalation is so full that it reaches the back of the lungs and causes the lungs to inflate laterally. This is actually called lateral breathing.

Contracting the abdominals, working the intercostal muscles between the ribs and breathing to the base of the lungs takes practice and patience. Correct breathing ensures strong blood flow to muscles, which energizes the body. Lastly, the muscles used in rolling and unrolling the spine, when doing Pilates exercises, opens and compresses the lungs naturally, thereby cleansing the lungs by forcing stale air out and allowing pure air in.

During every exercise, coordinated breathing, correct awareness of the body in motion, and alignment are emphasized.

CONCENTRATION

In a world that loves to multi-task, it's no wonder we have trouble concentrating. With the advent of technology, we are also experiencing an overabundance of pings and beeps from the different devices we rely on to keep our schedule, edit our documents, and stay in touch with friends and associates. By practicing the art of concentration and staying with one task to completion, you are reminding your mind and body that a commitment requires follow-through. Tenacity is a benefit that stems from healthy concentration skills. You will feel better, look better, and work better if you practice concentrating on one task at a time.

CENTERING

Finding your center is vital to achieving balance. Joseph Pilates coined the phrase "powerhouse" because the center is where all of our power is stored and converted to energy. Becoming aware of the power that is dormant in our core is the first step; using it for good is the second. Too many of us are unbalanced in our physical bodies. We subconsciously favor one part over another, leaving our bodies without a true center to guide us. *Once you find your center and cultivate its strengths, it will bring balance into every physical position and activity, including moments of rest.* It is important to note that if you train the body to work out of alignment, then you walk and function out of alignment. The converse is also true. **Practicing and exercising in alignment will create a strong, functional body.**

CONTROL

Maintaining control over your body and mind is crucial to your health. When we feel out of control, we also feel stress. Stress sets off a chain of unraveling physiological symptoms that can distract you from your goals. Keep your mind clear, your body strong, and your level of mental and physical control high. You will notice that when stress comes on, rather than internalizing it, you will be more apt to acknowledge it, breathe through it, and continue on. Easier said than done you're saying, but when control over your body and mind becomes second nature, your health will improve dramatically.

FLOW

Pilates loved to work with dancers because he could see the promise that stems from free-flowing movement. Imagine that your arms and legs are like a marionette's, hanging loose from your shoulders and hips as though suspended from strings. Let your limbs go freely into each movement; unrestricted by tension. Glide as you walk, allowing your heel, arch, and then toes to feel the floor with each step. Let go of the tension that limits the usefulness of your limbs and allow them to move without constriction from the joints they are attached to. Move as though each position is a chance to circulate the oxygen in your body.

FLEXIBILITY

Flexibility is vitally important to a longer, healthier life. Staying flexible means keeping your joints healthy and in good use. After all, **once our joints degenerate, they do not repair themselves.** Awaken the connection between the limb and connective tissue by stretching with the same intensity as you exercise. Most importantly, **stretch throughout your day.** If you have a few seconds, roll your neck, ankles and wrists. Any free moment is enough to move your body.

PRECISION

Pilates is not a difficult workout method to master. The exercises are very straightforward and easy to learn. However, *the restorative properties of Pilates are lost if the practice is not rooted in precision.* Each movement must be grounded not only in intention and breath, but also in a technical understanding of the desired goal. As you become more experienced in your Pilates practice, it becomes more important to understand the how and why of each exercise. After all without precision movement is often wasted.

ROUTINE

Finally, you are ready to incorporate all of these principles into a regular practice. By establishing your new Pilates-based restorative exercise routine, you are taking a first step to a longer, happier, and healthier life. However, like all good intentions, without following through, you will never meet your goal. **The best part about Pilates is that you can practice it anywhere, even on the go. Yet, it is the student who integrates their workout into their daily and weekly calendar that sees the best results.** Start off with only what you can handle, and then gradually build more workout time, as you are able. Starting off with great intentions but not enough commitment will only set you back over time. As you first begin to practice your Pilates workouts, reward yourself when you follow through; soon enough, you will find that working out is reward enough. **Consistency is key.**

GOOD POSTURE: GOOD HEALTH

If one performs Pilates mindfully there will be an intention and focus on the muscles. **When you train your body properly you will be much more aware of your positioning. You will sit taller, elongate your body and feel coordinated in motion.** Taking the time to "do Pilates" is a key to becoming more aware of your own biomechanics and will help prevent musculo-skeletal deficiencies and correct those already present.

Pilates will develop lengthened, flexible muscles that have greater strength, reducing the chance that muscle imbalances and overcompensation will occur.

The exercises must be done regularly and routinely. Don't be surprised, when in the very near future, you start reading more and more research about the benefits of Pilates and spinal pain management, both acute and chronic.

The body works as a unit and there must be a balance between the stabilizing muscles as well as the muscles of activity. Sitting incorrectly causes muscular overcompensation and ubiquitous weakness.

Balance, accord, harmony, body position and posture are fundamental to the Pilates Method. This is why each and every exercise emphasizes abdominal and spinal stability and gets to correct muscle imbalances and unnecessary forces on the joints and musculo-skeletal structures.

A WORD ABOUT ERGONOMIC CHAIRS

In a quest to alleviate back, neck and/or shoulder pain, many manufacturers make chairs that are ergonomically designed to minimize fatigue and improve both posture and productivity. If you are currently in a state of dysfunction, ergonomic chairs can be a lifesaver.

The chair supports weaknesses in your musculo-skeletal system, keep in mind, however, that nothing compares to your own strong body at work for a strong muscular system. <u>Movement is Key!</u>

Try not to sit too long. Take breaks often.

EVERY SPINE TELLS A STORY

Performing Pilates and improving spinal health will give you a heightened self-awareness. You will find that you will function in your movements with greater ease, endurance and strength. Moreover, if you have any physical ailments that impede you from fully functioning, you will find these will dissipate or may become completely eliminated with practice. Pilates isn't meant to be a cure-all, but in its own way it will improve how the body functions.

"In 10 sessions you will feel the difference. In 20 you will see the difference and in 30 you'll have a whole new body."

—Joseph Pilates

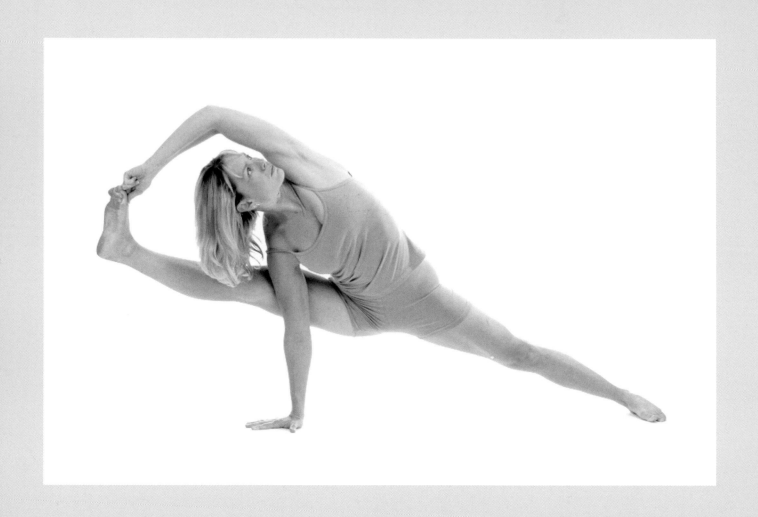

PART 4:

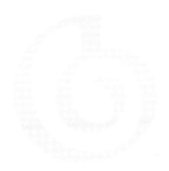

THE MINDFUL WORKOUT

BEGINNING BASICS

"Each muscle may cooperatively and loyally aid in the uniform development of all our muscles."

—Joseph Pilates

POSITION YOURSELF

Before beginning your Mindful Workout, there are a few concepts you should become familiar with. It will take you more than a few sessions to intuitively focus on each one, so remember to be patient and let your body think for you. These beginning basics will enhance the effectiveness of your workout.

FOOT POSITIONING

It is so important to pay attention to our feet, as any standing position relies on the balance achieved through proper foot positioning. Our feet have the awesome responsibility of supporting our entire body, which allows for locomotion and helps us maintain healthy posture.

THE EXERCISE

1. Stand with your feet shoulder width apart and parallel to each other.

2. Roll your feet inward onto the inner soles, then outward onto the lateral borders of the foot. Finally, find the center, where you feel your feet evenly balanced.

3. Lift all ten toes up, off the floor, and then place them down. Repeat this one more time and feel the toes evenly distributed, from the right pinky to the right big toe and the left big toe to the left pinky.

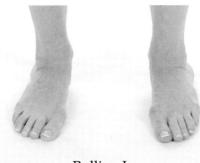

Rolling In

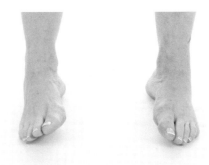

Rolling Out

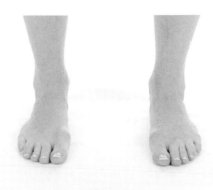

Balanced

FEET

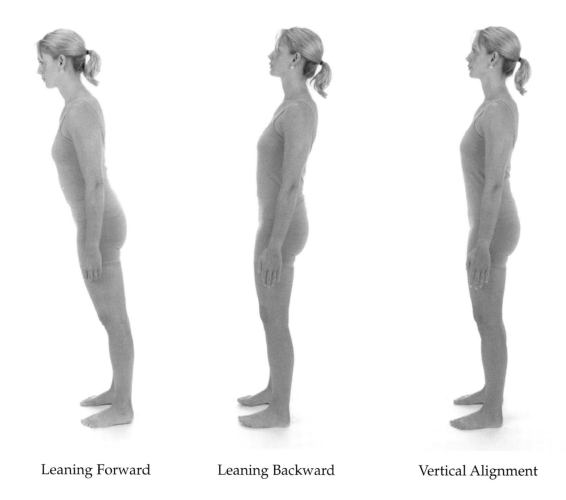

Leaning Forward   Leaning Backward   Vertical Alignment

Next, place some weight on the heels followed by the balls of the foot. Rock carefully back and forth to find a perfect balance between the two. Feel the weight of your body supported evenly by your feet.

PILATES STANCE

Pilates stance is really a misnomer, as it has little to do with foot position, but everything to do with aligning the legs so that you initiate the work from the base of your pelvis. While exercising, you should actually pay very little attention to your feet.

If you are a person who already walks turned out, then the stance should be very slight. If you are a person who walks slightly pigeon-toed, then the turnout position is vital. It's all about balance.

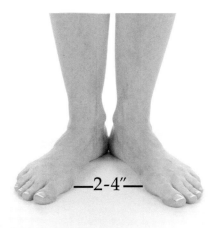

Stand with your toes about two to four inches apart and your heels together.

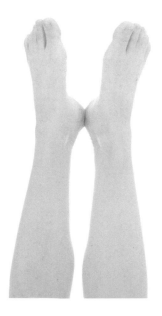

Pilates Stance

Foot position with legs in the air.

HELPFUL HINT

It is important to begin the Pilates Stance with your inner thighs. To see the difference, try engaging your inner thigh muscles as you move into Pilates Stance with your legs parallel and then with your legs turned out. You will feel the difference when your feet are turned slightly out.

THE SCOOP

The Scoop describes the action of pulling the transversus lower belly muscle into the spine and up toward the rib cage.

THE EXERCISE

1. Contract this girdle-like muscle to decrease your abdomen's diameter by bringing your navel towards your spine and gently up into your rib cage.

2. Next, imagine circling a corset around your rib cage to tighten the upper abdominal muscles, knitting the ribs together.

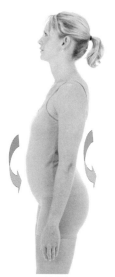
Loose Stomach Muscles

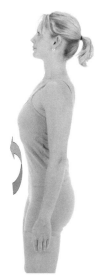
Breathing In To Pull The Stomach In

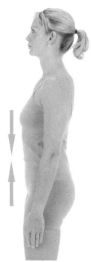
Contracting The Lower & Upper Abdominal Muscles

HELPFUL HINTS

☺ Try not to let the hip or shoulder joints move when tightening the lower belly muscle. You do not want to rotate the pelvic girdle under, nor roll the shoulders forward. Simply pull your navel to your spine and lift in and up.

☺ To feel the transversus abdominis: wrap your hands around the front of your hip and lower belly and cough. The tightening of the transversus protects the internal organs and supports the lower part of the pelvis.

VISUALIZATION

Imagine a flat ice cream spatula dredging through your favorite ice cream tub.

THE SCOOP

DO YOU KNOW YOUR NEUTRAL SPINE FROM YOUR NEUTRAL PELVIS?

Of course, the spine and pelvis are two separate anatomical parts. However, because one activates the other, it is often difficult to separate their individual functions during movement. Learning to isolate your neutral pelvis will improve the quality of your workout. Here's how:

1. Lie on your back and bend your knees and place your feet on the floor, hip width apart. Keep your buttocks relaxed and focus on your spine, independent of your hips. Place your index and second finger on top of your pubis bone and your palms on top of your hip bones. Draw your thumbs together about two inches below your belly button—Your hands should be configured in a triangle shape.

2. Tilt the pelvis as far back as possible, as if you were jamming your back into the mat and your pubis bone was pulling toward your nose.

3. Shift the direction of the pelvis, and lift the hip bones forward so the pubis bone goes to the floor.

4. Now, imagine you have a hot cup of tea, balanced in the middle of the triangle. Find the exact center point, so that the water would not spill into your belly, nor spill out between your legs. This is neutral pelvis and can be exhibited very differently on each person.

   For correct spinal alignment, lengthen the spine along the floor and feel a slight lift in the lower back (lumbar region) and behind the neck. This creates a neutral spine, with two natural curves, and should be noted in all the exercises.

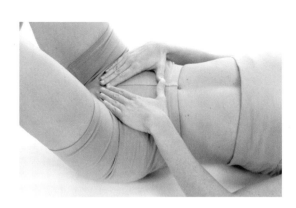

Neutral Pelvis

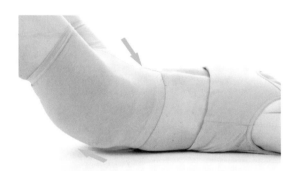

The lower back lifted off the floor.

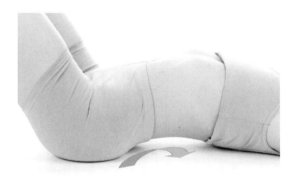

The middle back arched off the floor

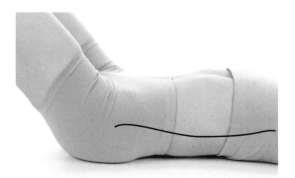

Neutral spine

SHOULDER GIRDLE MOBILITY AND STABILITY

For seated professionals who tend to lean or hunch in their seats, strengthening the stabilizing muscles of the shoulder blades can help prevent muscle fatigue, which can avert overuse conditions such as thoracic outlet syndrome or repetitive strain disorders.

THE EXERCISE

Gently pull your shoulder blades down towards your back ribs and then slightly together.

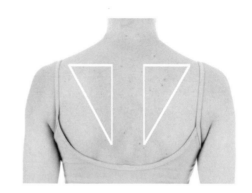

SEATED CONSIDERATION

This shoulder blade stabilization exercise will enhance posture, spine, and shoulder alignment.

TRY THIS!

Next time you are in your car, sit in your seat, with your lumbar region (lower back) into the backrest. Gently open your shoulders so they touch the edges of your seat and lift the back of your neck slightly. You will be awed by your posture! In addition, your outlook will automatically and dramatically improve. Add a smile! Tony Robbins calls this changing your physiology. It really does work!

HELPFUL HINT

Be careful not to jam your shoulder blades together, which over contracts the muscles between your shoulder blades. Instead, be mindful of broadening your upper back as you drape your shoulder blades along the back ribs.

CONNECT THE RIBS

Ribs sometimes "pop" up when you are lying on your back while simultaneously bringing your arms overhead. To create a connection, keep pulling your bellybutton into your spine while maintaining a neutral pelvis. This is very challenging.

THE EXERCISE

Keep the ribs connected by activating the abdominal muscles and the oblique side muscles of the trunk, pulling both in towards your midline.

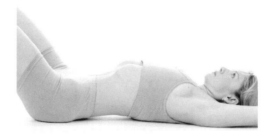

Ribs popping up

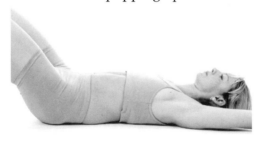

Keeping the abdominal wall of muscles
contracted and pulled together

VISUALIZATION

Imagine a child wanting to jump on your stomach and you need to protect it.

HELPFUL HINT

Don't go beyond the point in any exercise where you lose this abdominal contraction.

NECK LENGTHENING

It's important to reduce the stress on your neck and shoulder muscles.

When performing exercises that involve lifting your head off the mat, be mindful of a neutral neck position. Since our posture actually starts at the base of your skull, it is important to be aware of the entire length of your spine. As you gain strength and develop this awareness throughout the distance of your spine, end to end, these head-lifting exercises will become easier.

If you EVER feel pain or strain in your neck while performing Pilates exercises, rest your head for a moment. When you can, continue with the exercise with your head lifted or support the head with one hand.

INCORRECT NECK POSITIONS:

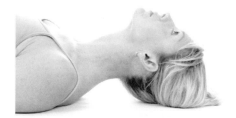

Too Long

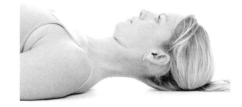

Too Short

TRY THIS!

An easy way to align the neck is to imagine holding an egg under your chin. If you pull the chin too close to the chest, the egg is crushed; on the other hand, if the chin is lifted too high, toward the ceiling, the egg will fall out. Find where the neck is neutral.

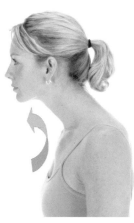

Too Forward

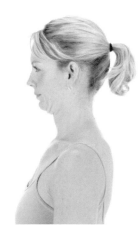

Too Backward

NECK POSITIONING WHEN ON THE MAT:

THE EXERCISE

Lift your head and bring your chin towards your chest. Look into the abdominals or ahead to maintain a neutral neck position.

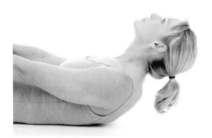

Too Opened

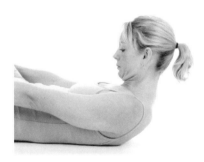

Too Closed

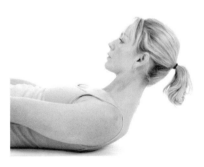

Just Right! Neutral Neck

"Above all, learn how to breathe."

—Joseph Pilates

LATERAL BREATHING

Joseph Pilates was asthmatic, therefore full breathing was essential to his work. He also knew, back then, as we do today, that inhalations cleanse the lungs and improve circulation and exhalations purify the bloodstream of noxious waste and toxins.

THE EXERCISE

1. Place your hands on your rib cage, over your lungs. Inhale completely through your nose, filling the lungs with air. Expand the ribs laterally, without lifting the sternum (chest plate). This is quite a challenge. Finally, exhale fully through your mouth.
2. Repeat for three full cycles.

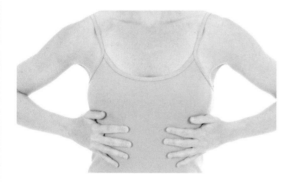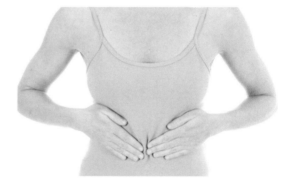

CHALLENGE

Imagine filling up only one lung at a time by placing one hand on the lung you are filling and the other hand at your side. This is a great mental exercise too!

VISUALIZATION

Imagine fully inflating and deflating a balloon.

HELPFUL HINT

Look in a mirror if necessary. Maintain an abdominal contraction so you learn to fill your lungs with clean oxygen, while simultaneously staying connected to your core muscles.

STRATEGIC STRETCHES
"PRE-PILATES STRETCHES"

The following Pre-Pilates stretches are foundational to a complete Pilates workout. Each isolates and supports a different area of the musculoskeletal system and can be performed in different variations.

Take the time to stretch routinely; you will experience less pain and enjoy life more, both in and out of the office.

ON YOUR MARK, GET SET, GO!

You've learned about the Pilates principles. You've learned about the impact Pilates can have on your body, your career, and your life. Now, it's time to put your intention to action. All you need is an exercise mat and comfortable clothing for these stretches and exercises.

Remember, each exercise has both a stretch and strengthen phase. Execute both with the same intensity and intention.

Breathe in, Beathe out, and Let's begin.

NECK

ALPHABET NOD:

To warm & stretch the neck muscles.

THE EXERCISE

Sitting or standing comfortably, use the end of your nose to trace the capital letters A through E in midair to loosen the cervical vertebra.

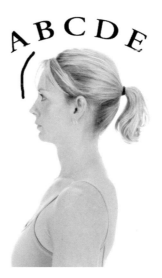

HELPFUL HINT

Alphabet Nod:

Larger letters will provide greater range of movement.

PAINT BRUSH:

To help identify a 'neutral neck'.

THE EXERCISE

1. Lie on your back, and bend your knees so they are shoulder width apart and your feet on the floor/mat. Put an imaginary paintbrush on the end of your nose and paint an imaginary vertical line on the ceiling with the brush.

2. Complete four "yes" nods.

HELPFUL HINT

Paint Brush:

If you drop your chin too far down, the imaginary paintbrush looses contact with the ceiling. The opposite occurs if the chin lifts too high. Keep the range of movement within normal limits.

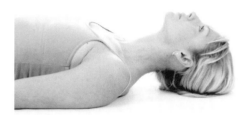
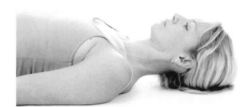

SUSPENDED BAGEL:

To loosen the upper cervical vertebra.

THE EXERCISE

1. Lie on your back, with your knees bent and your feet on the floor. Visualize a bagel suspended above your nose from a string on the ceiling. Outline the thickest part of the bagel with your nose to loosen the axis and atlas (two top) cervical vertebra.

2. Complete three rotations.

3. Change direction for three more circles.

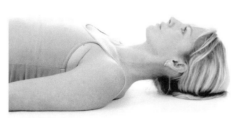

NECK

SHOULDERS

PUPPET ARMS

To isolate the shoulder blades and their placement on the back.

THE EXERCISE

1. Lie face up with your knees bent. Open your collar bones to expand your shoulders and back of the ribs. "Plug" the top outer corners of your shoulder blades into the mat imagining that you are making an impression.

2. Raise your arms to vertical, palms facing each other, and imagine that your hands are being suspended by marionette's string. Raise the right arm to the ceiling so as to lift the right shoulder blade off the mat.

3. Hold it for a second then bring the arm and shoulder blade down.

4. Lift the left hand and arm up to the ceiling and lower it, imagining the puppeteer guiding the hands up to the ceiling to lift and lower the shoulder blade.

5. Repeat right and left for four sets.

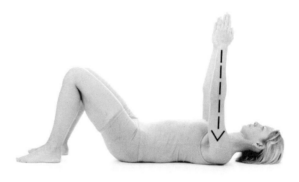

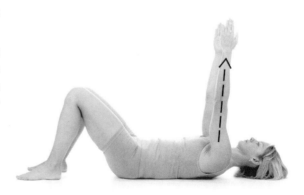

ELBOW CIRCLES

To open the joints & stretch the muscles of the shoulder girdle.

THE EXERCISE

1. Lie face up with your knees bent. Place your hands on your shoulders with your elbows kissing each other above your nose.

2. Draw both elbows down toward your belly. Then, open the elbows wide apart and bring them to the floor by your hips. Remember to keep your hands on your shoulders.

3. Scrape the floor with your upper arms and draw the elbows up above your forehead until they circle around to meet above your nose, elbows together.

4. Repeat four times and change directions for four repetitions.

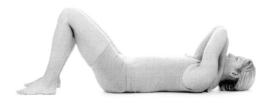

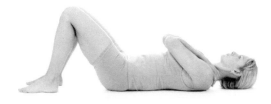

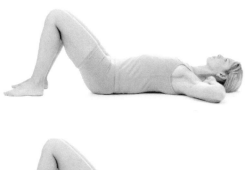

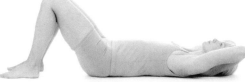

SPINAL ARTICULATION

To enhance mobility of the individual spinal vertebrae.

THE BRIDGE

THE EXERCISE

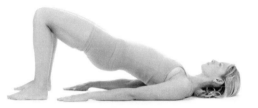

1. Lie face up with your knees bent, hip distance apart. Bring your arms down by your side, palms down. Elongate the spine and open your shoulders to imprint them into the mat. Gently pull in your abdominals.

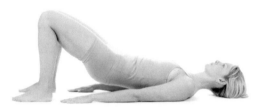

2. Lift your tailbone off the floor as you pull your pubic bone toward your nose and gently press your feet into the mat. Continue lifting until you have created a bridge from your shoulders to your tail, creating one straight line.

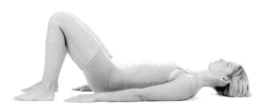

3. Roll down, from the upper back through the mid-back down to the tailbone.

4. Articulate up and down four times as you focus on mobility of each vertebra of the spine.

VISUALIZATION

Imagine that the bony protuberances of your spine are sprockets of a bike and you are laying them down into a chain that is on the mat. Be mindful that there is space between each sprocket and that the chain is straight.

HIPS & PELVIS:

KNEE LIFTS

To strengthen the hips & lower abdominal muscles.

THE EXERCISE

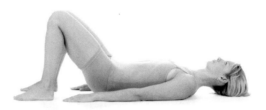

1. Lie face up with your knees bent, hip distance apart. With your arms down by your side, palms down, contract your lower abdominal muscles, by gently pulling your navel to your spine, without rotating your pelvic girdle under.

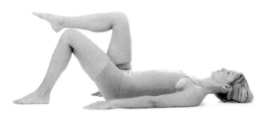

2. Bring the right knee up to 90° so that the knee is in direct line with the hip joint. Bring the left knee up to 90° and keep the knees hip distance apart. Continuing to keep the transversus (lower belly) muscle contracted, lower the right foot to the mat, then the left.

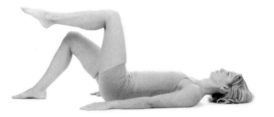

3. Repeat this lift and lower pattern, right knee and left knee, five times, slowly.

CHALLENGE

*   Bring both knees up at the same time and circle them together in one direction.
*   Switch directions, keep the back hips on the mat at all times.
*   Repeat three times.

This exercise truly targets the lower belly transversus abdominis muscle.

HIP JOINT STRETCH AND RELEASE & HIP CIRCLES

To isolate the hip socket and its surrounding tissues & release lubricating fluid.

THE EXERCISE

1. Lie face up with your knees bent. Draw both knees toward your chest so that the knees are directly above the hip joint, hip distance apart. Place your palms on the <u>front</u> of the thighs directly under the knees.

2. Inhale and press your hands into your knees, while resisting your knees with your hands. Hold for three seconds. Exhale to release. Repeat three times.

3. Next, place your hands <u>on top</u> of the knees, keeping the knees hip distance apart. Inhale and press your hands into your knees as you resist your knees into your hands. Hold for three seconds. Exhale to release. Repeat three times.

4. Place your hands on the <u>outside</u> of the knees, keeping the knees hip distance apart. Inhale and press your hands into your knees as you resist your knees into your hands. Hold for three seconds. Exhale to release. Repeat three times.

5. Place your hands on the <u>inside</u> of the knees, keeping the knees hip distance apart. Inhale and press your hands into your knees as you resist your knees into your hands. Hold for three seconds. Exhale to release. Repeat three times.

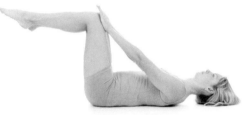

Hands on the <u>front</u> of the knees

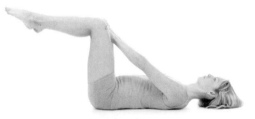

Hands on the <u>top</u> of the knee

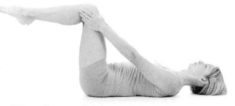

Hands on the <u>outside</u> of the knee

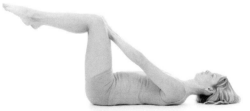

Hands on the <u>inside</u> of the knee

6. Now, place both hands on top of the knees and draw both knees into your chest, circle them apart, draw them together and bring them up toward the chest again, making circles with your knees.

7. Circle the knees three times and then change to the opposite direction three times. Be generous with the movement.

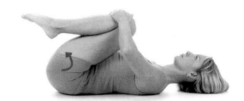

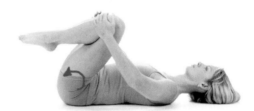

HELPFUL HINT

This exercise works because the force exerted by pressing your hand has an equal and opposite force on the other end of the thigh bone.

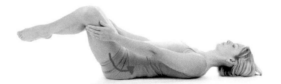

VISUALIZATION

Imagine a bowl of warm taffy and the back of a ladle pulling the taffy. Think of the taffy (ligaments) in the bowl (hip socket) being pulled (stretched) on the back of the ladle (top of the thigh bone). Then stir the bowl of taffy.

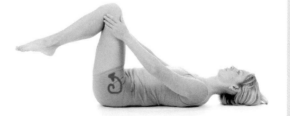

GENTLE LUMBAR RELEASE

To free up the lowest part of the spine.

THE EXERCISE

1. Lie face up with the knees bent, feet on the floor, hip distance apart.

2. Exhale to create an abdominal contraction and lift the tailbone and lower back slightly off the floor.

3. Contract the pelvic floor muscles by pulling in and up. Hold for 2 seconds.

4. Inhale and gently roll the lower spine down to neutral.

5. Repeat five times.

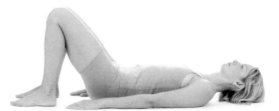

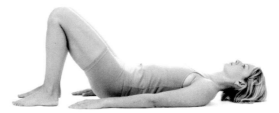

HELPFUL HINT

The most effective form of this stretch is to purely use the abdominal muscles to move the pelvis; that is, when the stomach muscles are contracted, the lower back muscles are relaxed allowing a stretch. Try not to use your thighs.

VISUALIZATION

Think of a hammock swinging freely.

LOWER BACK OPENER

To stretch the hamstring & lower back.

THE EXERCISE

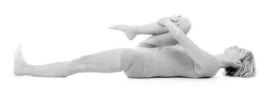

1. Lie on your back with one knee drawn into your chest and the other leg long on the floor, with your foot flexed (toes reaching to the nose).

2. Hold onto your knee with both hands, and stretch it to the chest. Hold to stretch the hamstring and lumbar region for five full breath cycles.

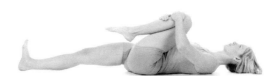

3. Switch knees and repeat the breathing.

VARIATIONS:

⑥ Bring both knees into the chest & hug them in.

⑥ Bring the knee towards the armpit (along the side ribs) for a deeper stretch.

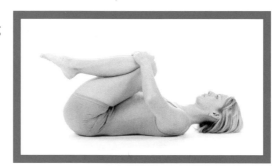

HELPFUL HINTS

⑥   With each breath, pull further to the chest, while simultaneously lengthening the opposite leg.

⑥   Hold under the back of the thighs if you have knee concerns.

LOWER SPINE RELEASE

To open the lower back, hips, waist & shoulders.

THE EXERCISE

1.   Lie on your back with your knees bent, feet on the floor. Bring your arms out to the side, making a "T".

2.   Slowly exhale and draw both knees over to the right side, allowing the knees to come as close to the floor as possible without creating tension in the spine. Inhale and exhale as you fall farther into the stretch.

3.   Inhale again and exhale to bring the bent knees over to the left side. Breath consciously to stretch further. Again, inhale to prepare and exhale to bring the legs up and over to center. This exhaling is important as it causes the abdominal muscles to contract which protects your back.

4.   Repeat the sequence three times.

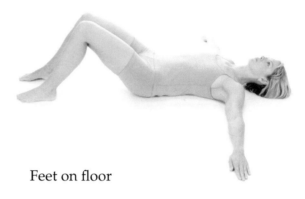

Feet on floor

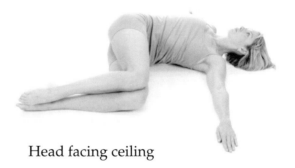

Head facing ceiling

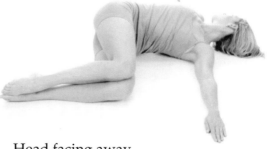

Head facing away

1. Bring your knees up to 90° like a tabletop with the feet off the floor and the arms out to the side. Turn your head to the opposite direction of your knees.

2. Bring one leg straight down onto the mat while bending the opposite knee to the chest. Draw the knee over to the opposite side. Turn the head to the opposite direction of the bent knee.

CHALLENGE

Try to maintain shoulder contact while bringing the knees to the floor.

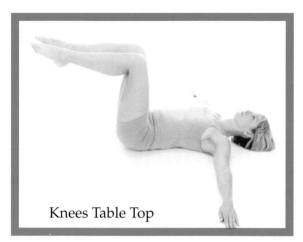

Knees Table Top

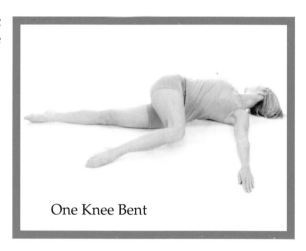

One Knee Bent

LOWER BACK

SITTING HAMSTRING AND BACK STRETCH

To stretch the back of your legs and spinal muscles.

THE EXERCISE

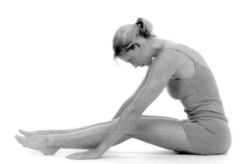

1. Sit on your bottom of your sit bones. Moving the flesh away from your bottom while seated is helpful. Sit taller and lengthen your spine longer. Extend your legs long in front of you, parallel to the hips.

2. With the arms on the floor by your sides, exhale and stretch your torso toward your thighs. Hold for ten counts and release up on an inhalation.

3. Repeat four times.

HELPFUL HINTS

⑤ To simplify the exercise, simply bend one knee to the side to stretch one leg at a time.

⑤ To ease tight muscles during this exercise, bend the knee slightly.

⑤ At home, you can stretch one leg at a time by placing it straight on the edge of a bed & the other leg dangling off to the side. Stretch toward the lengthened leg.

HAMSTRINGS

VARIATIONS

1. Hollow out the abdominal area and gently tuck your tail under to lengthen your spine to open the lumbar region of your lower back. Imagine a "C" in your spine, with the strongest curve at the lumbar region.

2. With the chest toward the thighs, reach for the feet, drawing the crown of your head toward your toes.

3. With the chest toward the thighs, lift the sternum (chest plate) up and try to flatten the lower abdomen to the top of the thigh, while pulling the toes back toward the shins.

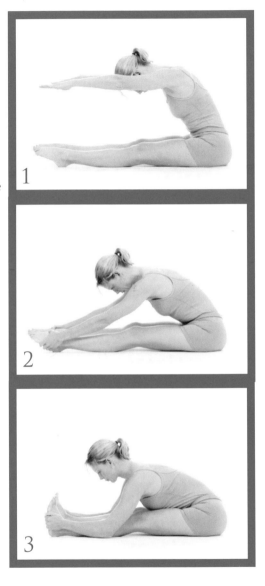

THE QUADRUPED: ON ALL FOURS

THREAD THE NEEDLE

To stretch the shoulder, neck, upper back and arm, one side at a time.

THE EXERCISE

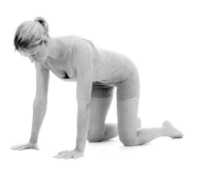

1. Kneel on all fours with the hands directly under the shoulders, and the knees directly under the hips, shoulder- and hip-width apart.

2. Inhale and lift your left hand out to the side and up toward the ceiling. Stretch the chest and muscles.

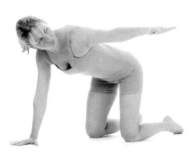

3. Exhale as the arm descends and needle it under the supporting arm until you float down to your left shoulder.

4. Let the head and neck relax. Inhale in the stretch and exhale to further the stretch. Inhale again as you float your arm back up to the ceiling. The breath simply facilitates the stretching.

5. Repeat four times on one side, then the other.

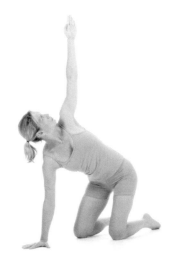

Bring the arm forward long in front of you, while pressing the same side hip away from your midsection. Create a "smile" with your side before threading the arm.

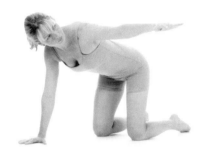

VISUALIZATION

Imagine your arm being a needle and you are threading it through the opposite side opening.

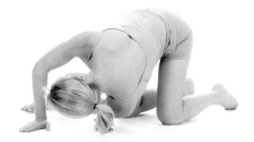

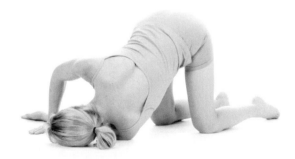

BACK

CAT STRETCH

To open & close each vertebrae, which nourishes the spinal column as well as stretches the muscles between the back ribs.

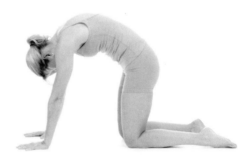

THE EXERCISE

1. Kneel on all fours with a neutral spine and place your hands directly under your shoulders, and your knees directly under your hips, shoulder-and hip-width apart.

2. Inhale to prepare and exhale as you tuck your chin to your chest.

3. Tilt your tail under toward your knees. Round your back up to the ceiling as if you were a scared cat.

4. Exhale and release the spine to neutral.

5. Repeat for three full cycles.

VARIATION

For further spinal articulation, you may repeat the above exercise, while lowering the belly toward the floor and slightly lifting the head and tail to create an arched back. This generates less disc space between the vertebra and releases more lubricating fluid in the joint space. (Do not do this variation if you have a weak or vulnerable back.)

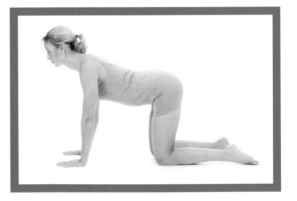

VISUALIZATION

Think of a wickedly scared cat

SPINE STRETCH

62

ALL 4'S SWIMMING

To strengthen the muscles between the vertebrae, the shoulders & hips and also challenge your balance.

THE EXERCISE

1. Kneel on all fours with a neutral spine. Place the hands directly under your shoulders, and your knees directly under your hips, shoulder-and hip-width apart. Gently contract the abdominal muscles for support.

2. Inhale and extend the right arm and left leg in opposition to each other, making an "x" with your arm and leg.

3. Exhale as you hold the pose for five seconds. Return to the starting position.

4. Repeat with the opposite arm and leg and hold for five seconds. Repeat 5 times each leg and arm.

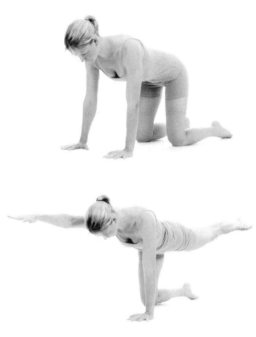

VARIATIONS

1. Perform with only the legs, keeping the knee facing the floor and the toes long.

2. Perform with only the arms, keeping the arms straight (without locking the elbows) and the fingers reaching long. Your hand position can either be facing the floor or in a Karate chop position.

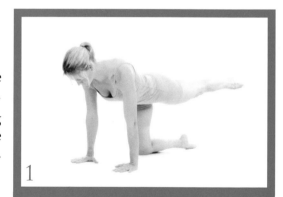

1

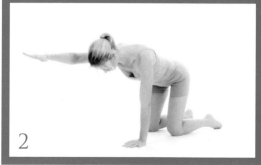

2

HELPFUL HINTS

☉ The core must be engaged in all the variations.

☉ Variations should be performed <u>first</u> if All 4's Swimming is unstable.

ERECTOR SPINE EXTENSION

To strengthen the muscles of the back that help support the spine.

THE EXERCISE

1. Lie face down, resting your forehead on the floor. Place your arms down by your sides, palms facing up.

2. Inhale and lift your head, heart, and arms up. Continue lifting as the crown of the head ascends and the chest lifts off the floor.

3. Hold for three seconds. Exhale as you descend to the floor.

4. Repeat five times.

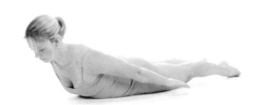

VARIATION

1. Place your hands under your forehead, to make a little pillow. Lift the crown of the head, elbows and chest off the floor, maintaining a triangle with the arms.

2. Hold for five seconds and release slowly.

3. Repeat five times.

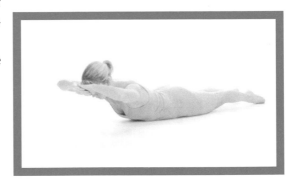

VISUALIZATION

Lengthen the neck and imagine lifting your head to where the ceiling and wall meet, where crown molding might be placed.

SWIMMING

To strengthen the arms, legs & back, while improving coordination & control.

THE EXERCISE

1. Lie face down, arms and legs extended long. Contract the abdominals by putting an imaginary grape under your belly button.

2. Inhale and lift your head and right arm, as high as possible. Alternate raising your arms with vigor.

3. Inhale and exhale for three cycles. Rest.

4. Perform with just the legs.

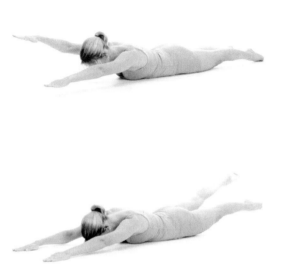

VARIATIONS

⑥ Perform with just the right side (arms and legs) and hold for 5 seconds. Repeat for the left side.

⑥ For a challenge, lift both arms and legs and flutter both extremities.

⑥ Lift your head "out of the water."

REST POSE
(Also known as child's pose)

THE EXERCISE

1. Sit on your knees and shins with your abdomen still slightly contracted. The forehead is on the floor. Place your arms beside your legs.

2. Rest in this pose and breath effortlessly, but mindfully.

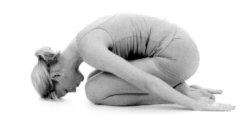

VARIATIONS

1. Place your arms straight above your head, and rest your hands on the floor.

2. For a further spinal stretch and release, you may open your knees and let your abdomen lie between your thighs.

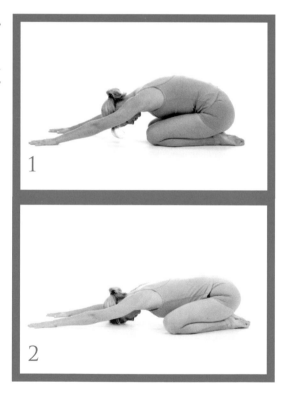

THE
EXERCISES

THE EXERCISES

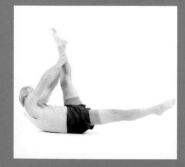
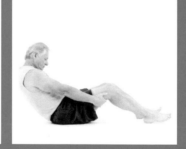
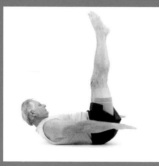
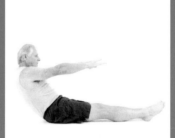

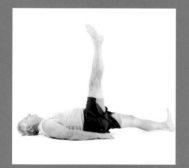
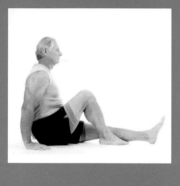
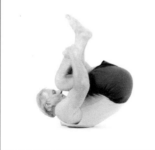
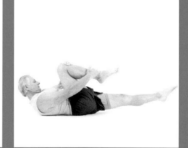
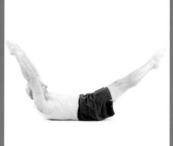

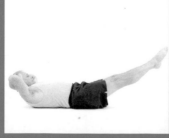
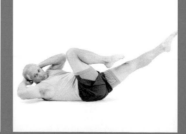
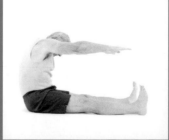

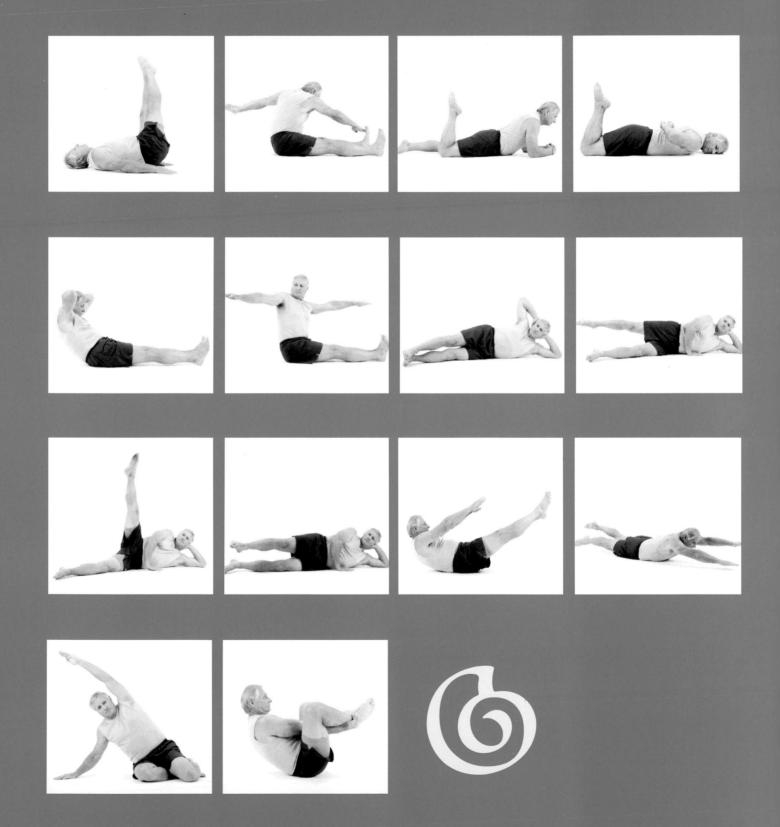

THE EXERCISES

As you move into The Exercises, you will begin the journey of understanding your own mind-body connection. Do them to the best of your ability, but mostly enjoy the process.

"You are as old as your spine is flexible."

— Joseph Pilates

CONSCIOUS CONCEPTS:

Generally, whenever the body is bending or flexing, such as when the chest moves towards the thighs in a crunch sit up, there is an exhilation. Knowing this, you can trust that eventually your breath will fall into rhythm with your movement. Don't think about the breath so much that it gets in your way.

⟳ Remember, each exercise has both a stretch and strengthen phase. Execute both with the same intensity and intention.

"Where your eyes go, the body follows."
—Juli Kagan

⟳ If you look at your core when doing an exercise, the energy of the movement will go into the core. Conversely, if you look up to the ceiling, for example, your neck muscles will be strained, placing undue stresses on other joints, muscles and body parts.

⟳ In <u>all</u> exercises where you are lying on the floor, draw your shoulder blades down your back, elongate your spine and contract your abdominal muscles in and up. Maintain a neutral pelvis and neutral spine. Mastering this position is a challenge; be patient.

⟳ Finish every exercise feeling as though you could stand up, breathe deeply, and walk out of the room ready to present yourself. To do this, always be mindful of your motion and position while executing the exercises.

GETTING READY

You've learned about the Pilates principles. You've learned about the impact Pilates can have on your body, your career, and your life. Now, it's time to put your intention to action.

THE EXERCISE

1. Stand with your feet in Pilates stance. Lift your toes off the floor, and then place them down, feeling all ten toes evenly balanced on the mat. Gently feel your heels on the floor and equilibrium between the front of the foot and the back of the heel. Imagine there are roots growing down into the earth pulling the base of your feet down.

2. Gently press your ankles and calves together.

3. Gently press your knees together, so that if a piece of paper were put between the knees, it could be pulled down. Zip up your inner thighs, and gently press them together.

4. Think about lengthening your tailbone down to the floor without rotating your pelvic girdle backwards. Keep your pelvis in line with the pubic bone.

5. Pull your navel towards your spine, and imagine bringing your belly button up and into your rib cage. Gently engage your abdominal muscles by shortening the distance between your lowest rib and the top of the hip bone. From your ribcage down you should be about 25% contracted.

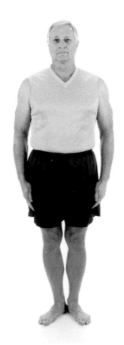
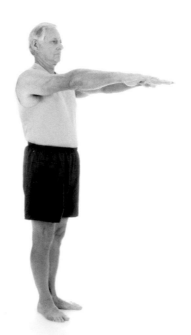
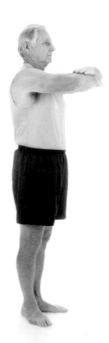

6. Check that your collarbones are parallel to the floor and perpendicular to the chest-plate.

7. Bring your chin slightly toward your chest, as if you were holding a small apple or egg.

8. Cross your arms into a "genie position."

9. Cross one foot in front of the other.

10. Sit down with balance, trying to do so without your hands.

11. Once on the mat reach the hands down and move yourself to the middle and lie down.

VISUALIZATION

Imagine your head is filling with helium. Lift your spine up through your crown towards the ceiling.

TRY THIS!

To double-check that you are able to connect to your Powerhouse, try this pre-workout move:

Lie down and pull your knees into your chest. This opens up your lower back. Make a ball with your body lifting your head, neck, and shoulders. Let the weight of your stomach muscles sink down into the back of your spine. Gently squeeze your abdominal muscles in toward your midline. Feel the contraction.

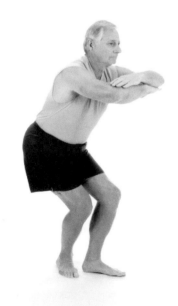
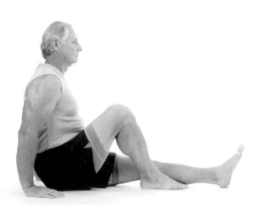

THE HUNDRED

The Hundred was designed to increase circulation and warm the body in preparation for the rest of the matwork, so it is always performed first in the Pilates workout. The Hundred coordinates breathing and heart rate with movement, by generating deep breaths that help circulate blood flow and build stamina. You will literally feel your body get warm as you vigorously pump the arms and challenge the breath.

THE EXERCISE

1. Lying face up on a mat, bring your knees into your chest.
2. Pull your navel gently into your back and strongly up into your ribcage.
3. Lift your head and look into your belly.
4. Reach your arms long by your thighs.
5. Stretch your legs up to the ceiling in Pilates stance.
6. Pump the arms up and down, at the height of your abdominal wall.
7. Inhale to a count of 5 and exhale to a count of 5.
8. Repeat 10 cycles until you have done "100" breaths.

VISUALIZATION

Imagine a balloon expanding and deflating, to improve circulation.

For the challenge: Imagine a bowling ball going down your legs, like a slide, landing in your belly, to improve strength.

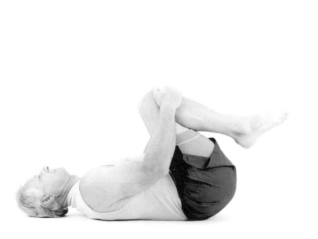
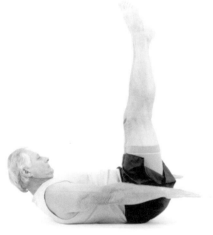

CAUTION

- If your neck gets fatigued at any time, rest your head on the mat. When you are ready, lift it back up and continue. Keep doing the exercise, even when your neck is inactive.

- For lower back care, keep the knees bent at a 90° angle, like a tabletop.

- If your hamstrings (back thigh) muscles are tight, keep your knees bent.

CHALLENGE

- Lower your legs until they are 45° from the mat. Be certain your lower back remains flat on the mat.

- Keep reaching your middle fingers towards the feet. You should have your arms long and shoulders down.

- Keep the base of your shoulder blades on the floor. Imagine the weight of your feet, plus the weight of your head sinking into your abdomen. Now, put that imaginary egg under your chin. As you gently grip the egg, focus your eyes toward your abdominal muscles.

SEATED CONSIDERATIONS

The Hundred strengthens the torso, which helps prevent back injuries from improper seated posture. The 100 can improve your lung capacity and oxygen consumption making you feel more vital.

TRANSITION TO NEXT EXERCISE

Draw your knees into your chest and lower your head.

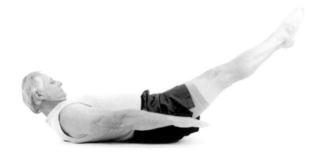
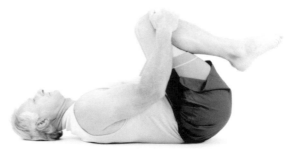

THE HUNDRED

ROLL DOWN

The roll down helps you learn how to connect to your powerhouse.

THE EXERCISE

1. Start from an upright seated position, with your knees bent. Roll your back down toward the mat, gently holding onto the back of your thighs for support.

2. Curl yourself up, looking into your navel. Try to create a "C" curve in your spine as you bring your chest to your thighs.

3. Repeat 8 times.

VISUALIZATION

Imagine yourself getting up and over a heavy bowling ball that is cradled in your lower abdomen.

CAUTION

⊚ Avoid lifting your shoulders to your ears; use the muscles of your powerhouse.

⊚ Do not use momentum to help you up! The work is in pulling your navel in and up toward your ribs and spine.

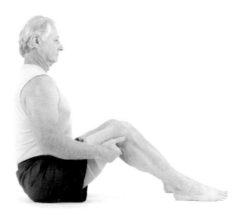 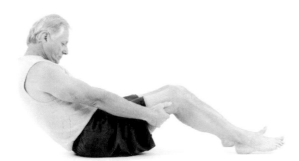

CHALLENGE

    ♢ Slow the movement down considerably and use full control.

    ♢ Pull your abdominal muscles deeper into your midline, initiating from the lowest abdominal muscles.

    ♢ The lower you roll down, the more challenging to get back up.

SEATED CONSIDERATIONS

This exercise prevents seated back injury by strengthening abdominal muscles and creating a supple spine.

TRANSITION TO NEXT EXERCISE

Lie on your back.

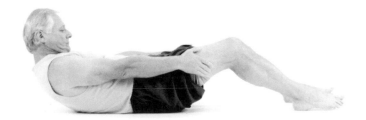

THE ROLL UP

The Roll Up emphasizes abdominal strength, while stretching the spine extensors and hamstrings (back of the thighs).

THE EXERCISE

1. Straighten your legs all the way down the mat, and squeeze the backs of your thighs together.

2. Bring your arms up toward the ceiling, and then float them back to a high diagonal. Imprint your spine into the mat while you stretch so as to not allow the back to lift off the mat, nor allow your ribs to pop up.

3. Initiating from your core muscles, bring your chin towards your chest and peel your back off the mat, "rolling up" and over toward your toes. This takes great strength.

4. Stretch over towards your toes, and bring your chest to your knees. This is the stretch phase. Simultaneously, keep your navel pulled back toward your spine, as if you were pregnant. Reach forward, but pull back in the waist, working in opposition.

5. Smoothly roll back towards the mat, squeezing your inner thighs and keeping your arms parallel, reaching towards the toes. Feel your lower, then middle, and finally your upper back roll down the mat.

6. Bring your head down last, and reach your arms up toward the ceiling, while still imprinting your spine into your mat. Float the arms back again, maintaining that imprint of your spine.

7. Repeat 5-8 times.

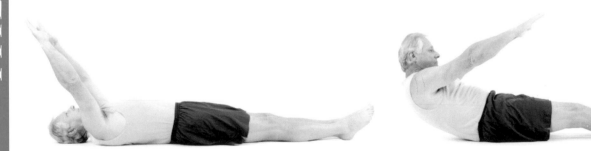

BREATH

Inhale: Reach your hands up and back to a high diagonal.

Exhale: Roll up and stretch towards your toes.

Inhale: As you reach toward your toes.

Exhale: As you lower each vertebra down, bone by bone.

VISUALIZATION

Imagine a magnet pulling your chest and arms forward toward your legs. Then imagine the magnet resisting your pull, as you roll back down.

CAUTION

✆ If you have a hard time with this "roll up," bend your knees slightly, with your feet on the floor, bring your hands under your thighs to help you to a sitting position.

VARIATION

Individuals who have a vulnerable back or weaker abdominal muscles should "Roll-Down" only. See page 76.

TRANSITION TO NEXT EXERCISE

Draw your right knee into your chest, and stretch it up to the ceiling, while holding onto either your calf or hamstring. Lengthen your left leg down onto the mat.

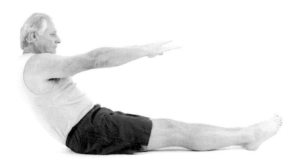
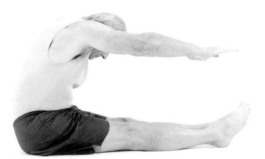

LEG CIRCLES

Leg Circles strengthens the hip, promotes release of lubricating fluid in the joint and stretches the hamstring and side of the upper leg.

THE EXERCISE

1. Stretch your right leg up towards the ceiling, and focus on stretching your hamstring. Flex and point your toes for added stretch, while holding your calf.

2. Rotate your leg slightly to the right.

3. Bring your hands down to the mat, and pull your navel into your spine.

4. *Imagine you have four large screws securing the bones of your shoulders and hips into a wooden floor beneath you.*

5. Lengthen the back of your neck, gently feeling your shoulders on the mat.

6. Bring your right foot toward your left shoulder and over towards the left arm. Stretch your upper thigh. Keep your right hip on the mat.

7. Circle your leg around and down toward your toe, then up toward your shoulder. Maintain your back against the mat.

8. Repeat in this direction five times, and then in the opposite direction five times.

   To transition to the other leg: Bring your knee into your chest, and draw your foot toward your other foot on the mat. Bring your left leg into your chest and repeat the stretching and leg circles.

BREATH

Inhale: Your leg crosses over your thigh and reaches down toward your opposite toes.

Exhale: Bring your leg slightly around and up to your shoulder.

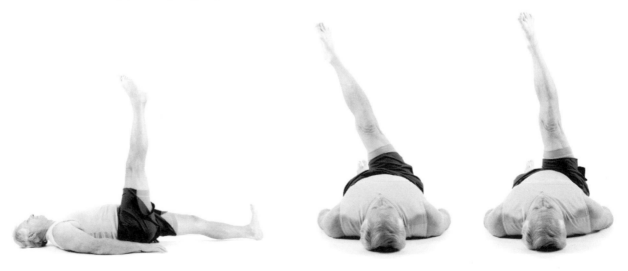

Stretch phase: Leg over thigh.

Strength phase: Leg comes around and up to your shoulder.

VISUALIZATION

Trace an oval shape on the ceiling, like a football.

CAUTION

- Keep your shoulders down and neck in alignment. (Hold onto an imaginary egg under your chin.)
- Use control to move your leg, not momentum.
- Start with small circles to gain control.
- If your hip clicks, keep your foot turned out and make the circles smaller.

CHALLENGE

- Make larger circles with your extended leg, but keep your hips fixed.
- Flex the foot on the floor for added stretch.
- Keep your navel drawn in and up further. Hug your midline.
- Pull your back onto the mat with strong stomach muscles, then lift the leg towards the shoulders.

SEATED CONSIDERATIONS

This exercise truly works the upper thigh and "saddlebag" area, most beneficial for those professionals who sit a large part of their day. Perhaps most important, it refreshes tired legs by increasing circulation.

TRANSITION TO NEXT EXERCISE

Bend your knees and squeeze them together. Bring your chin to your chest and roll your back off the mat, and come to a sitting position. Your hands can be under your thighs or on your shins.

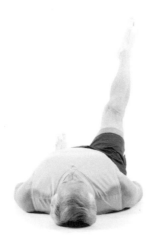

ROLLING LIKE A BALL

This exercise massages the spine and internal organs, while also improving abdominal control and balance.

THE EXERCISE

1. While sitting on your bottom, pull both knees into your chest.
2. Bring your knees up to your shoulders, keeping your heels together. Balance on your "sit bones" while holding your shins or ankles with your hands. Lower your head and look between your knees, noticing the distance between your heels and bottom. Try to maintain this distance throughout the exercise.
3. INHALE and roll back to your shoulder blades. EXHALE and roll up to your bottom, without letting your toes touch the floor. Balance! Mostly, try to maintain the integrity of the ball throughout the execution of the exercise by pulling your navel up into your spine.
4. Repeat the exercise 8 times.

CAUTION

◉ If you roll back to your head you have gone too far. Keep the chin tucked looking at your navel.

◉ Hold under your thighs, and open your knees, to create a larger ball which will facilitate an easier rolling action.

VISUALIZATION

For this exercise, think of the shape of a crescent moon or the action of a rolling ball.

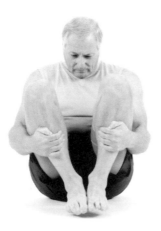 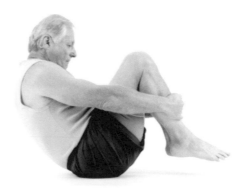

CHALLENGE

⚬ The closer your feet are to your bottom, the more challenging the exercise.

⚬ Cross your hands over your shins to make a smaller ball.

⚬ Pull the knees all the way up to the shoulders and tuck your head, to create the smallest ball possible.

⚬ Keep your shoulder blades down, especially as you come up to a seated position.

⚬ Keep the core engaged so as to maintain a "C" curve in your spine.

SEATED CONSIDERATIONS

This exercise challenges your balance, which is important for professionals who sit precariously on moving chairs with casters. It also promotes shoulder stabilization, especially helpful for those who hunch. Mostly, Rolling Like a Ball releases body tension.

TRANSITION TO NEXT EXERCISE

Place your feet on the mat, and place your hands next to your hips. Lift your hips up and back until your legs are straight. Roll back onto the mat, one vertebra at a time.

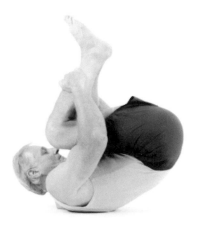
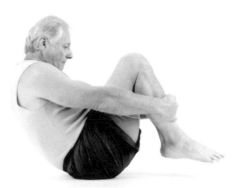

THE SERIES OF 5:

SINGLE LEG STRETCH

DOUBLE LEG STRETCH

SINGLE LEG STRAIGHT

DOUBLE LEG STRAIGHT

CRISS-CROSS

Ideally, the series of these five exercises are linked together, flowing from one exercise to the next.

The series can be performed independent of the entire workout, for those in a time crunch (pun intended). Alone, these exercises will improve your abdominal strength ten-fold. Do them daily!

The abdominals truly get a "massage" with this series. Your coordination will be challenged, but keep pushing through the entire repertoire. You will get stronger over time and soon enough, feel fantastic and accomplished!

SINGLE LEG STRETCH

The Single Leg Stretch simultaneously stretches and strengthens the legs while working the powerhouse.

THE EXERCISE

1. Bring your right knee to your right shoulder, and hold your right ankle with your right hand and your right knee with your left hand. This hand position helps keep the knee in alignment with the shoulder and hip. Do not pull in such a way that this alignment is jeopardized.

2. Lift your chin towards your chest, and lift your chest with your abdominal muscles. Look at your belly button throughout the exercise.

3. Draw your left leg into the chest then extend it out to a 45° angle. Strap your abdominals down.

4. Switch legs and change back to the right leg. Each time your knee comes into your shoulder, the same side hand goes to your ankle and the opposite hand goes to the knee.

5. Repeat five sets.

BREATH

Inhale: pull in the right then left knee.

Exhale: pull in the right then left knee.

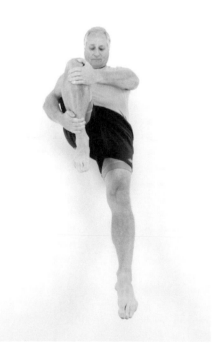
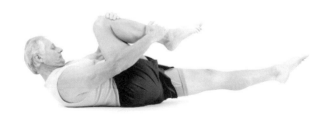

VISUALIZATION

Imagine that your back is glued to the mat and your legs are moving in line like pistons.

CAUTION

- If at any point you need to rest your head on the mat, do so, but bring it back up as soon as you are ready.

- For a weak back, keep your extended leg towards the ceiling, and keep your lower back on the mat at all times.

- For bad knees, hold under your thigh and do not pull in tightly.

CHALLENGE

- Lower your extended leg toward the floor, while maintaining a flat box.

- Press your spine further into the mat as you change legs.

- Maintain abdominal compression throughout the exercise, to prevent your body from rocking.

SEATED CONSIDERATIONS

This exercise stabilizes the torso, which prevents back injury and stretches the hamstring.

TRANSITION TO NEXT EXERCISE

Draw both knees into your chest and hold onto the shins.

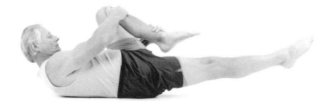 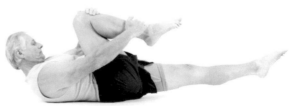

SINGLE LEG STRETCH

DOUBLE LEG STRETCH

This exercise stretches the body long and works the core, like never before!

THE EXERCISE

1. Place one hand on each shin, and hug your knees into your chest. Stay in a tight ball. Keep your head lifted while looking into your midline.

2. INHALE and reach your arms up and back to a high diagonal, keeping your upper arms glued next to your ears. Simultaneously extend your legs out to a 45° angle, and stretch yourself long as you compress your back into the mat. Keep your eyes focused on your inner thighs.

3. Squeeze your inner thighs from your tail. Make a trapezoid figure with your arms and legs, while reaching in opposition. Remain immobile as your arms and legs become secondary to the stability of your powerhouse.

4. EXHALE FULLY and swing your arms around and pull your knees in tightly to make a ball. Hug your chest to your thighs and stretch the lower back while sinking the navel into the spine.

5. Repeat the exercise five times.

VISUALIZATION

Imagine two people pulling your hands and feet away from each other simultaneously.

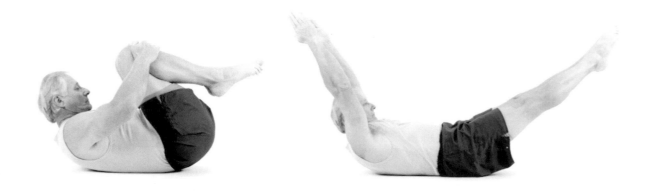

CAUTION

- ☙ For back concerns: Keep your legs higher to the ceiling.

- ☙ For knee concerns: Hold under the knees.

- ☙ For shoulder concerns: Keep your arms by your ears, so as to not hyperextend the arm at the shoulder.

CHALLENGE

- ☙ Lower your legs towards the floor while you stretch your arms and legs away from each other, as long as the back remains on the mat.

- ☙ Draw your abdominal muscles more towards your midline, while lengthening your sides simultaneously, to deepen the powerhouse.

- ☙ Place your hands lower on the shins, toward your ankles, to get into an even tighter ball.

SEATED CONSIDERATIONS

This exercise enhances back flexibility, develops stronger abdominals and improves breathing and lung capacity, allowing you to sit longer with poise and improved posture.

TRANSITION TO NEXT EXERCISE

Hug your chest to your thighs and stretch the lower back while sinking the navel into the spine.

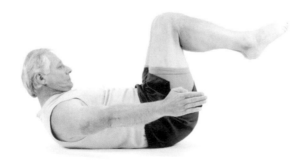 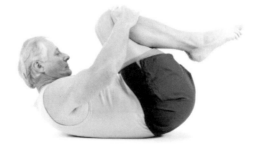

DOUBLE LEG STRETCH

SINGLE LEG STRAIGHT

The Single Leg Straight, also known as "scissors", stretches the back of your legs while continuing to strengthen your core interior.

THE EXERCISE

1. Bring your right leg up to the ceiling and hold the ankle with both hands.
2. Extend your left leg down to the mat, to about a 45° angle.
3. Lift your head and focus on your powerhouse.
4. Pull your navel into your spine, and *pretend there is a heavy weight on top of your stomach* that you have to hold tight in order to protect your internal organs.
5. Pull your right leg, which is straight, to your right shoulder. Pulse it further to the right shoulder with a dynamic movement. Energetically scissor-switch the opposite leg. Catch the other ankle and pulse it to the left shoulder twice. Open your elbows wide as you pull your leg in to gain arm strength.
6. The emphasis is on the powerhouse creating stability, even though the legs are moving vigorously. Bring the legs to your hands; that is, don't reach for your leg.
7. Pull the right leg and then pull left leg, repeating the exercise for five sets.

BREATH

Inhale: Pulse the right leg twice, and switch legs.

Exhale: Pulse the left leg twice.

VISUALIZATION

Imagine opening and closing scissors. Focus on the rhythm.

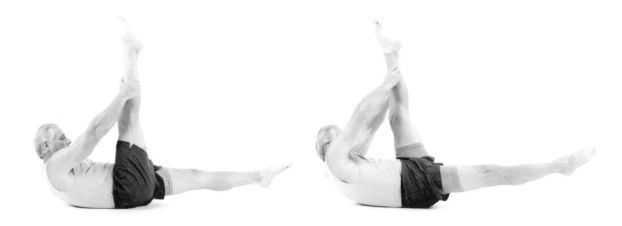

CAUTION

- If your hamstrings are tight, and you cannot reach the ankle, hold behind your hamstring or calf, keeping a bent knee.

- Keep your neck long and the shoulders relaxed. If the neck becomes fatigued, rest it from time to time, but keep working the powerhouse.

- Do not bounce or rock your body as you switch legs. Use the powerhouse to move them.

- Reduce the size of the scissor kick if you are inflexible.

CHALLENGE

- Reach the bottom leg longer to the mat.

- Quicken the pace of the switch, as long as you have control and coordination.

- Keep lifting your upper back off the mat throughout the exercise, coming to the base of the shoulder blades. Keep your knees as straight as possible.

- The most advanced challenge: Place your arms two inches above the mat, reaching long towards your toes as you scissor switch.

SEATED CONSIDERATIONS

This exercise stabilizes the trunk and increases hamstring flexibility.

TRANSITION TO NEXT EXERCISE

Bring both hands under the back of your head. Do not interlace the fingers, as this cuts off circulation. Gently rest the head in the hands but keep the abdominals activated. Keep looking into your powerhouse.

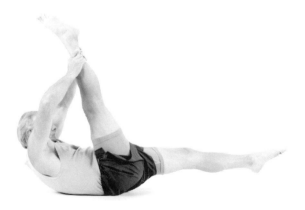

DOUBLE LEG STRAIGHT

The fourth exercise in the Stomach Massage Series, the Double Leg Straight, also called Lower and Lift, thoroughly challenges the powerhouse and core muscles.

THE EXERCISE

1. Straighten your legs up toward the ceiling and support your head with your hands. Continue focusing on the powerhouse; where you direct your attention is where the focus of the exercise will occur.

2. Initiating from the inner thighs, INHALE and lower your legs slowly about 18 inches, then EXHALE to bring your legs back up to the ceiling.

3. Repeat 5-10 sets, going lower with each repetition.

VISUALIZATION

Imagine a magnetic force resisting the legs down and controlling the legs up.

CAUTION

⊚ For a fragile back, place your hands (palms down) under your tailbone to support the lower back or bend your knees slightly in order to maintain your lower back on the floor throughout the exercise.

⊚ Do not lower the legs more than 1 inch at a time as they descend. Stay still in your torso. Work from the powerhouse; don't force your legs to go lower than necessary.

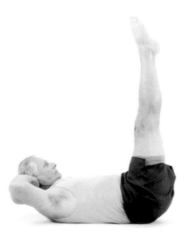
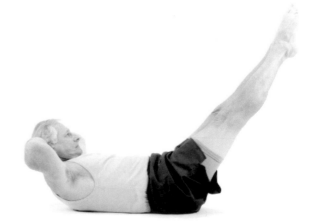

HELPFUL HINTS

○ *Maintain your shoulders and hips on the mat at all times.*

○ *Keep your stomach flat and your chin toward your chest.*

○ *DO NOT WORK FROM THE THIGH MUSCLES. Use your powerhouse to execute the exercise. If necessary, bend your knees a bit to relieve thigh fatigue.*

○ *If you are "stuck" in your thighs, try this: With your legs up toward the ceiling, tighten your thighs only, lower down 3 inches, and bring them back up. Do this two times. Now, release the contraction in the thighs, and put all the contraction in the core. From this posture, execute the exercise. You will really feel the difference between being in your thighs and being in your powerhouse!*

CHALLENGE

○ Change the rhythm of the exercise by emphasizing the down OR the up. The breath exhales on the exertion, lifting the legs up toward the ceiling.

○ Super Challenge: Lower your legs all the way down towards the floor! Just make sure your lower back stays on the mat.

○ Keep your shoulders down and your elbows wide.

○ Count three to lower the legs and one to lift the legs. Change the emphasis after five repetitions.

○ Make sure the legs do not go past 90° when they come back. This takes control and practice.

SEATED CONSIDERATIONS

This exercise truly works the lower powerhouse, ultimately supporting the lower back. It also focuses on controlled movement.

TRANSITION TO NEXT EXERCISE

Bend your knees into a table top position.

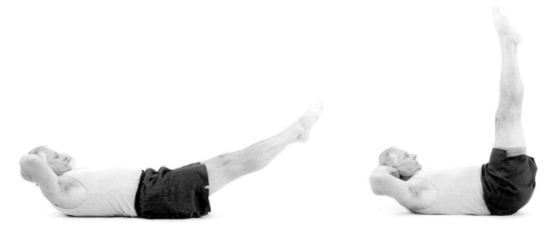

CRISS-CROSS (OBLIQUES)

The Criss-Cross strengthens the sides of the torso and whittles the waistline.

THE EXERCISE

1. Bend your right knee in line with your shoulder; extend the left leg out about 18 inches above the mat.
2. Bring your left elbow to your opposite knee.
3. Keep your back elbow lifted off the mat and look toward it. "Where your eyes go, your body will follow."
4. Change to the other side, "criss-crossing."
5. Keep reaching back to the rear elbow, lifting and turning from your oblique trunk muscles. Hold the lift, hold the twist, and hold the reach. Hold! Then switch. Slower is harder!
6. Repeat for 5 sets.
7. End by bringing your chest straight up toward your thighs-hold!

BREATH

Inhale: Twist to both sides.

Exhale: Twist to both sides.

VISUALIZATION

Imagine a hook hanging from the ceiling. Lift your elbow onto it.

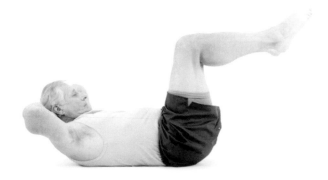
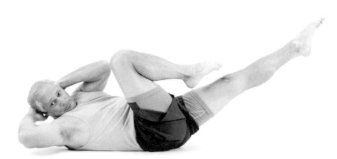

CAUTION

- Lift your chest to perform the crisscross; this is not a shoulder exercise, where the elbows flap back and forth.

- For lower back trouble or weak abdominal muscles: keep the feet on the mat with knees bent and twist only slightly until more strength is developed.

- Twisting should be avoided by anyone who has recently had a back injury.

CHALLENGE

- Maintain a deep abdominal contraction throughout the exercise.

- Reach your back elbow to the middle of the mat behind you.

- More challenge: Keep your knees bent like a tabletop, and work only the upper torso, leaving the legs still...Lift!

SEATED CONSIDERATIONS

Crisscross strengthens and improves spinal rotation, a movement that is often done when rotating on a wheeled chair in a small office space.

TRANSITION TO NEXT EXERCISE

Hug both knees into your chest and lower your head to the mat then lengthen both arms and legs long as if you were getting ready to dive into a swimming pool. Stretch your abdominal muscles.

Bring your arms and legs up to the ceiling and open them to a "V". Like a rag doll, roll up to a sitting position, feet and legs apart in a pie shape.

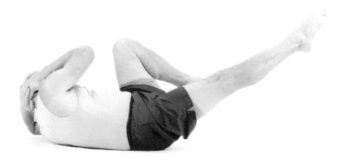

SPINE STRETCH FORWARD

This exercise opens the vertebral spaces that house the discs between the vertebrae, which contain spinal lubricating fluid. It also opens the muscles of the back and lengthens the hamstrings.

THE EXERCISE

1. Sit tall on your sit-bones with your legs a bit wider than your hips. Flex your feet up to the ceiling. Keep the middle toe in line with the knee, which should be in line with the hip. Keep it in a straight line while doing the exercise.

2. Bring your arms up so they are parallel to the floor in front of you. Sit taller. Grow "higher" *as if you were sleep walking.*

3. INHALE deeply to prepare for the stretch, then EXHALE and lower your head in between your arms, as the crown of your head reaches down toward the floor. Keep pulling your navel into your spine, lifting it up. Think about keeping your collar bones over your hip bones to create a "C" curved spine.

4. When you have exhaled completely, roll your spine back up bone by bone, imagine a zipper closing and INHALE fully. Come to where you started, sitting tall, as if your back was pressing against a wall.

5. Repeat 5 times.

VISUALIZATION

When the spine is stretching forward, envision going up and over a big beach ball. When the spine is lifting up, imagine stacking blocks one on top of the other, edge-to-edge and corner-to-corner.

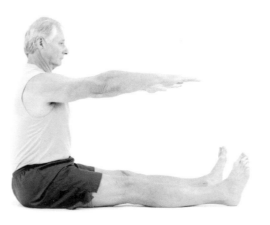 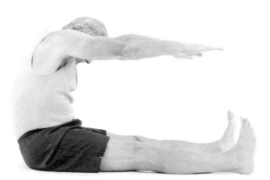

CAUTION

- ⊚ Keep your shoulders from lifting as you go up and over.

- ⊚ For back or flexibility concerns: bend your knees.

CHALLENGE

- ⊚ Gently squeeze your buttocks as you reach your hands to your toes. This pulls the tail down and lengthens the lower spine considerably, stretching it out.

- ⊚ Flex your toes throughout. This further stretches the back of your legs.

SEATED CONSIDERATIONS

This exercise particularly stretches the back and hamstrings, two areas vulnerable to tension and tightness.

TRANSITION

Bend your knees and bring them together about six inches from your bottom. Reach your arms forward, drop your chin toward your chest and slowly lower your back down to the mat, bone by bone. Use control; do this slowly.

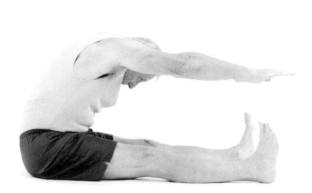
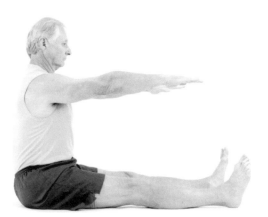

CORKSCREW

The corkscrew will help you gain control and strength of the powerhouse, especially the waist muscles.

THE EXERCISE

1. Place the palms of your hands on the mat beside your hips, for reinforcement.

2. Draw both knees into your chest and then lengthen the legs up towards the ceiling. *Imagine a belt keeping your the hips locked down.*

3. Make a slight "v" with your feet and gently squeeze your inner thighs to create a wrapping sensation toward the back of your thighs.

4. Circle the legs together beginning to the right, *as if you were drawing circles on the ceiling*, the size of dinner plates. *Imagine your toes holding a pencil.*

5. Stop at the beginning point and circle the legs in the opposite direction, pulling the legs towards your nose to start. Maintain your shoulder blades on the mat throughout the exercise.

6. Repeat 3 complete sets.

BREATH

Inhale: As the legs go around and away.

Exhale: As the legs come around and up toward the nose.

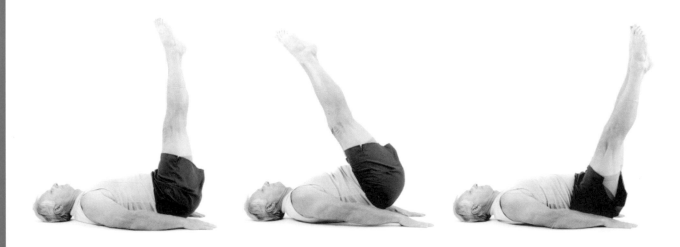

VISUALIZATION

Imagine balancing a stack of books on your abdomen-they are heavy and must stay balanced. Keep the ankles together with imaginary duct tape.

CAUTION

- ☙ Do not arch your back.

- ☙ Avoid any pressure on the upper cervical, neck vertebra

CHALLENGE

- ☙ Before beginning the circles, pull the knees and legs straight up to the nose first, and then circle around.

- ☙ Lift your hips off the mat when the legs elevate up and over your head. Be sure you are in control.

SEATED CONSIDERATIONS

The corkscrew especially targets the lowest belly muscle, the transversus. This girdle like muscle is one of the main stabilizers of the abdomen, necessary for strength and prevention of the "pooch" many women experience. It also greatly stretches the hamstrings.

TRANSITION TO NEXT EXERCISE

Bend both knees into your chest and lower your feet down to the mat. Come up to a sitting position as you perform the roll up with bent knees.

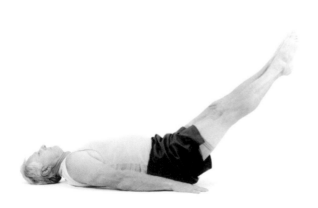
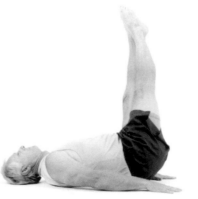

THE SAW

The Saw is like Spine Stretch Forward, but in a lateral, side direction. It works three things at the same time: the waistline, the hamstrings and breath. Opposition is the focus here.

THE EXERCISE

1. Open the legs until they are hip width apart. Align the toe, knee and hip and maintain them in one straight line.

2. Open your arms to the side so they are shoulder height and reaching long. Sit tall and make your back as long as possible, *as if a marionette puppet string was holding the crown of your head.*

3. Twist your body to the right and reach the opposite arm to the right. Exhale and "saw" off your pinky toe, with your pinky finger just outside the toe, going further and further with three small stretches. Keep the powerhouse engaged.

4. Inhale and stay twisted as you lift your back up. Untwist, sitting tall in your original position.

5. Repeat to the opposite leg.

6. Complete 4 sets.

BREATH

INHALE deeply and turn to the toe.

EXHALE all the air out of your lungs as you twist to the knee.

INHALE as you untwist, sit up and align your spine.

VISUALIZATION

Imagine that your sit bones are screwed down into the mat, while your thighs and calves are strapped down. The arms feel like taffy being pulled in opposite directions.

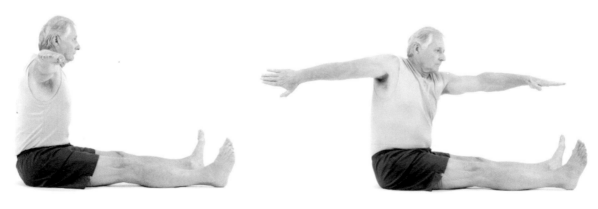

HELPFUL HINTS

⚕ Keep the hips stationary; that is, do not lift off the hip to reach further.

⚕ This is a breathing exercise; completely exhale all of the air out of your lungs as you reach for the toe. Inhale as you sit up tall.

⚕ Work the arms in opposition, with the back palm facing inward and upward.

⚕ Slowly stretch the hamstring as you keep the opposite hip on the floor.

⚕ Don't go for just a forward stretch over the knee. Pay most attention to the opposite hip placement and the lower back of the side being stretched.

CAUTION

⚕ If your hamstrings are tight, bend your knees to stretch as you reach.

⚕ Do not bounce to get further into the stretch, breath into it instead.

⚕ Keep the neck in alignment, turning the opposite ear toward the knee, if needed.

⚕ Do not lift the back straight up; articulate it up, *like a bike sprocket going into its chain.*

CHALLENGE

⚕ Work fully on opposition, lengthening, articulating and completely wringing the stale air out of the lungs- all simultaneously.

SEATED CONSIDERATIONS

Of the entire repertoire of Pilate's matwork, the Saw is one of the best exercises for the seated professional as it focuses on hamstring flexibility, and spinal rotation and mobility. These two areas of the body are the most physically abused by professionals who sit for long periods of time.

TRANSITION TO NEXT EXERCISE

Turn onto your stomach.

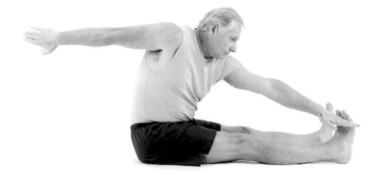

SINGLE LEG KICK

The Single Leg Kick strengthens the hamstrings, upper chest and back and stretches the front of the thigh.

THE EXERCISE

1. Prop up onto your elbows and make a fist with one hand and draw the other hand around it. The forearms are flat on the mat. If you looked down, you would see your arms in a circular configuration.

2. Lift your chest up *like a sphinx* and pull your elbows back towards your hips so you stay erect in your back and abdominal wall. This is the hard part of the exercise-to stay lifted with your shoulder blades draping down your back.

3. Lengthen the legs long and hold them together at the inner thighs. Toes are toward the floor.

4. INHALE and bend the right knee toward you bottom twice, with a lively pace.

5. Switch to the other foot before the right foot goes down towards the floor. EXHALE and kick the buttocks twice. Alternate the breath with the kicks.

6. Repeat 5 sets.

VISUALIZATION

Imagine a turtle coming out of its shell; neck long, chest proud.

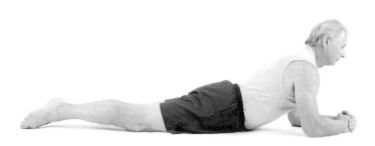

CAUTION

- For bad knees: decrease the range of bending or leave it out completely if you feel discomfort.

- Do not sink into your shoulders-keep pulling your elbows towards your hips to help you stay lifted in your chest.

- Kick with energy, but maintain a contact with the pubic bone and thighs on the mat. Think of rotating the pelvic girdle under slightly so your buttocks doesn't rise at all.

- Keep the legs together to initiate contraction of the inner thigh muscles.

- Keep the abdominals lifted and elongated.

CHALLENGE

- Focus on coordination, flowing movement and pace of the leg switch.

- Try to kick the foot all the way to the buttocks.

- Don't let your feet hit the floor during the exercise.

SEATED CONSIDERATIONS

The Single Leg Kick strengthens the hamstrings, upper chest, and shoulder stabilizing muscles. This helps you to sit more erect and proud.

TRANSITION TO NEXT EXERCISE

Lay down on the mat with your cheek to one side for the Double Leg Kick.

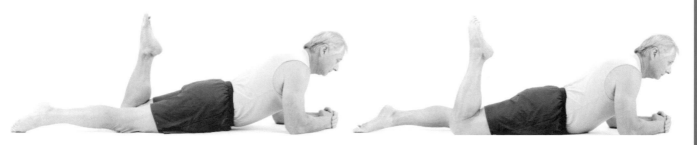

SINGLE LEG KICK

DOUBLE LEG KICK

The Double Leg Kick stretches the shoulder girdle and chest and strengthens the hamstrings and back.

THE EXERCISE

1. Extend your legs long. Hold both hands together, one on top of the other, at your tail and glide them up towards the middle of your shoulder blades, as high as possible. Allow the elbows and shoulders to fall open.

2. Gently squeeze your inner thighs and bottom muscles, while anchoring your hipbones into the mat.

3. INHALE and kick your feet simultaneously to your bottom three times without lifting your hips. EXHALE and extend the legs back to the mat and stretch your arms to your feet, as you lift your upper back.

4. Continue reaching your clasped hands to your feet and lengthen your spine.

5. Return your chest to the mat and turn to the opposite cheek.

6. Bring your hands to your upper back to begin another cycle, being mindful of the pace and energy of your movements.

7. Complete 2-3 sets.

BREATH

Inhale: Kick the feet three times.

Exhale: Lift the chest and extend the arms.

VISUALIZATION

Imagine being Kate Winslet, when she is lifting her chest and face to the wind, while Leonardo DiCaprio, is supporting her back, in the movie: Titanic. Be proud, lifted and hold the position.

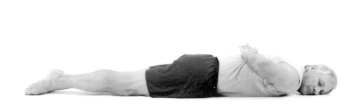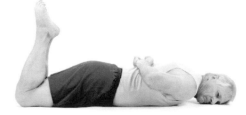

CAUTION

- Do not do this exercise if you feel pain in your shoulders, back or wrists.

- To make the exercise easier on the shoulders, do not hold the hands. Simply keep the arms by your sides, with your hands facing your thighs.

- Protect your back by keeping your navel pulled in and up.

CHALLENGE

- Bring your hands as high up as possible between your shoulder blades at the start of each repetition.

- Hold the chest up for an extra count.

- Move more slowly and deliberately throughout the exercise.

- Keep your feet on the mat behind you as you lift up.

- Elongate your body, from the crown of your head to your toes.

- Change the breath, inhaling on the lift.

SEATED CONSIDERATIONS

This is an excellent exercise for the seated professional who regularly sits with a rounded back. This exercise opposes and reverses that position. This exercise is also especially helpful for spinal flexibility and strength.

TRANSITION

Come onto all fours and bring your buttocks over to your heels. Rest for a moment. Allow the lower back to stretch but don't loose your abdominal contraction; keep the powerhouse slightly lifted off your thighs. Come onto your back for the Neck Pull.

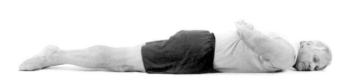
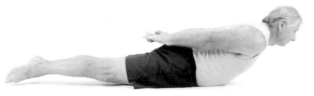

NECK PULL

The Neck Pull is one of the most challenging abdominal strengthening exercises. Do your best!

THE EXERCISE

1. Lying flat on the mat, stretch your legs long and place them shoulder width apart. Flex your toes back.

2. Place your hands, one on top of the other, behind the nape of your neck. Let the elbows open towards the mat.

3. Start by lifting your head up and looking toward your feet, then peel your back off the mat, vertebra by vertebra, making a "C" curve in your back. Bring your head over towards your knees, keeping your navel in and up, *as if a ball were in your belly.*

4. Slowly, lift your back up straight and tall, opening the elbows back and wide.

5. With control, curl your back down, slowly, bone by bone. Squeeze your tail gently, to facilitate a stretch in your lower back.

6. End with the elbows flat on the mat and the head relaxed in the hands. Work the exercise with rhythm and not momentum.

7. Repeat 5 times.

BREATH

Inhale: To prepare.

Exhale: As you peel your back off the mat.

Inhale: To sit tall with elbows wide.

Exhale: Rolling your spine down slowly: lower, middle, and finally upper back.

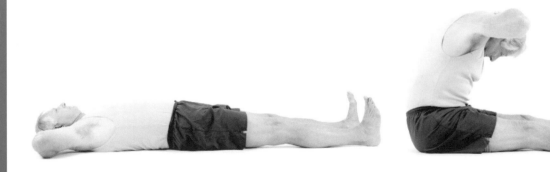

VISUALIZATION

Come up like a fishing line pulling in a heavy fish.

CAUTION/MODIFICATIONS

- ☙ Do not jerk or use momentum to get up.

- ☙ If this arm position is too challenging at first, then work with the hands under the thighs to help transition the back up to a seated position

- ☙ Place your hands at the back of your head, and cradle your head so the elbows come together in front of your nose. Then roll up toward your thighs.

- ☙ Place the hands together at your forehead.

CHALLENGE

- ☙ Keep the back flat as you descend back toward the mat behind you. Look to the horizon. Hinge back until your abdominal muscles can no longer hold on or your feet start to come off the floor. Then, bring your chin to your chest and roll back.

SEATED CONSIDERATIONS

The Neck Pull is the quintessential abdominal strengthening exercise. A strong front yields a supported spine, vital for the seated professional.

TRANSITION TO NEXT EXERCISE

Roll up to a seated position, legs long and together.

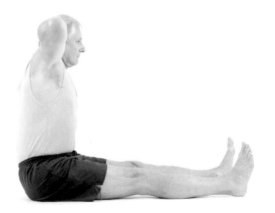
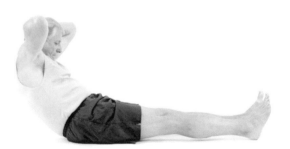

SPINE TWIST

Spine twist trains the trunk to spiral on the vertical axis of your spine; while maintaining a stable pelvis. It is also a breathing exercise where you completely exhale all the "stale air out of your lungs" as Joseph Pilates would say.

THE EXERCISE

1. Flex your feet and lock them together, keeping your hips and legs glued to the floor. Open your arms as wide as possible.

2. Sit tall on your sit bones with a very straight back.

3. INHALE to prepare and EXHALE as you twist to one side, lifting from your waist.

4. Pulse two times going deeper into the stretch on the second pulse. Keep pressing your heels together.

5. INHALE and rotate to the center, continually lifting your chest, lengthening your back and pulling your lower abdominal muscles in and up.

6. Twist to the other side.

7. Repeat 3-5 sets.

VISUALIZATION

Imagine a lid being taken off a jar: it is lifted as it is twisted, but the base must stay solid.

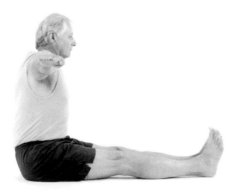 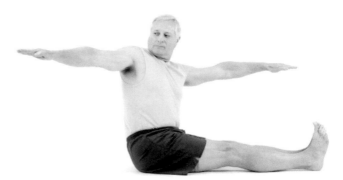

CAUTION

- This exercise can be challenging. Stay within a range of movement that is healthy.

- For shoulder concerns: you can bend the back elbow as you turn.

- Do not reach the arms out of your vision, especially by swinging them forcefully; use control and work slowly.

CHALLENGE

- Work extra slowly.

- Look beyond your back hand and go further. Feel the arms work in opposition, all the way to your fingertips.

SEATED CONSIDERATIONS

The Spine Twist will enhance hip and waist flexibility, as well as release the spine. Mostly, it will work the muscles that support your back, allowing you to sit tall. This exercise will create a heightened awareness of your posture in general.

TRANSITION TO NEXT EXERCISE

Lie down onto your left side and align your back against the back edge of the mat.

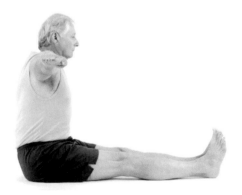
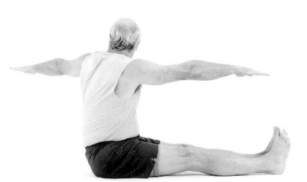

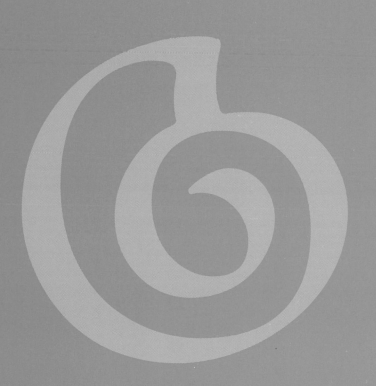

SIDE LEG SERIES:

FRONT/BACK
LIFT/LOWER
SMALL LEG CIRCLES

The Side Leg Series enhances hip joint mobility, strength, stability and muscle tone. It is completed on one side before changing to the other.

THE EXERCISE

1. Lying on your left side, align your shoulders, back and hips with the longer, back edge of the mat.
2. Prop your left elbow onto the mat, and place your left hand next to your ear.
3. Place the right hand in front of the chest, acting like a seatbelt for control.
4. Lift both feet off the mat simultaneously, and bring them to the front corner of the mat.

VISUALIZATION

You would look like a boomerang if you took a picture from the ceiling.

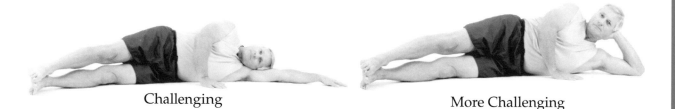

Challenging   More Challenging

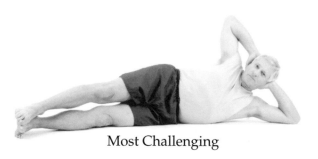

Most Challenging

FRONT/BACK

THE EXERCISE

1. Lift your top leg two inches above the bottom knee. Keep this leg parallel to the floor, at this height, throughout the exercise. For a variation, you can turn the knee up to the ceiling.

2. Kick your foot towards your nose, keeping it as stretched as possible. Pulse it two times at the furthest point.

3. Draw your leg behind you, and reach it long towards the opposite position. Keep your body in alignment while stretching and reaching your leg as far as possible in both directions.

4. Repeat 5 times.

VISUALIZATION

Imagine kicking over a bowling pin that is placed three feet in front of your nose. Reach for it!

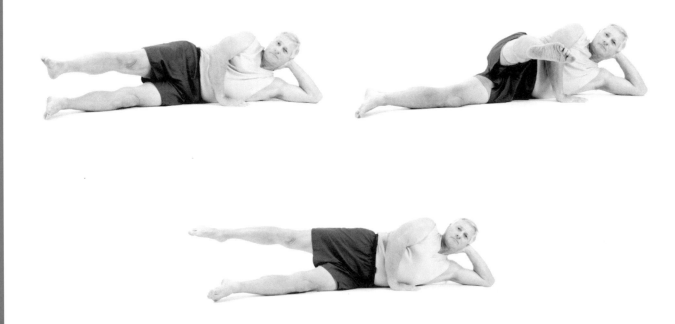

LIFT/LOWER

THE EXERCISE

1. Turn your knee up to the ceiling slightly. Keep your powerhouse strong, and do not move your shoulders or hips.

2. Lift your leg up to the ceiling with control.

3. Lengthen your leg slowly down to the floor with power and resistance. Invite your mind to help you focus on this work.

4. Lengthen from your waist, encouraging your foot to reach longer than the bottom leg. Do not use momentum to lift the leg. Lift your leg up like a feather and press it down sturdily-defying gravity.

5. Repeat 8 times.

VISUALIZATION

Imagine your leg being stretched like taffy as it comes down.

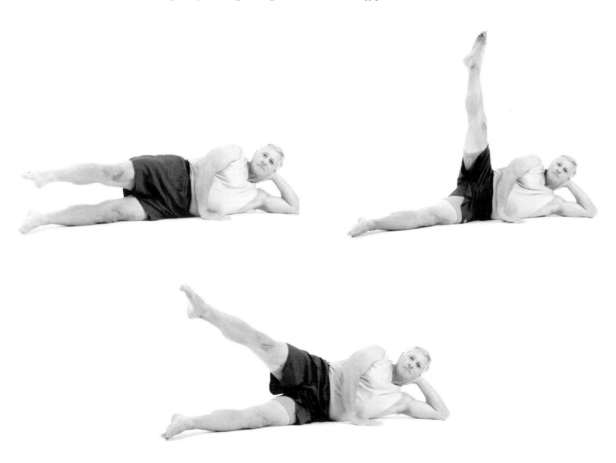

SMALL LEG CIRCLES

THE EXERCISE

1. With a fully extended leg, circle your leg around, imagining you are drawing a circle on the wall beyond you, with your toe reaching all the way from the hip joint.

2. Make the first four circles the size of a dinner plate and make the next four circles the size of teacup. Keep your motion small if you are rocking.

3. Reverse direction after eight complete circles.

VISUALIZATION

Imagine someone pulling your leg out of your hip socket to make it longer.

Keep your hips and shoulders in alignment by imagining that you have a dowel or curtain rod going from the ceiling through your hips and shoulders, and then down into the floor beneath you.

Imagine a pencil on the end of your toe, and you are drawing circles on the wall beyond you...Remember the point gets dull, so you must keep reaching further as you progress.

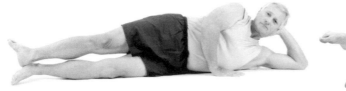 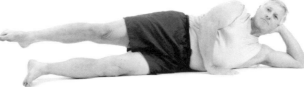

CAUTION

- Do not look down at your feet; keep your neck long.

- Swing your legs with control. Do not use momentum to see how far you can kick.

- Do not reach the leg so far behind you that it causes strain in the lower back. Make your movements small and defined.

- Stay stable in your pelvis. No rocking toward your back or belly.

CHALLENGE

- Bring the hand forward to the side of your head.

- Keep your leg parallel to the height of your hip, as well as to the floor, as you kick forward and back.

- Think length not width to create a long, strong muscle.

SEATED CONSIDERATIONS

For women, the leg series is the antidote for thick thighs, which are a side effect of too much sitting and not enough moving. For men, this exercise strengthens the hips and gluteal muscles, both important muscles for seated posture.

TRANSITION TO NEXT EXERCISE

Roll onto your back.

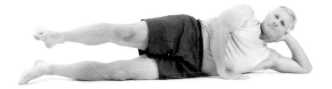

THE TEASER *(The supreme Pilates exercise)*

Of all the Pilates moves, The Teaser truly measures abdominal control and strength.

THE EXERCISE

1. Bring your knees into your chest.

2. Bring your arms and legs up to the ceiling. Turn your feet out slightly so you can engage your inner and back thighs. Plug your shoulders into your back.

3. Lift your head and lower your legs to a 45° angle. Control your abdominal muscles by sinking your navel into the mat.

4. INHALE and reach your arms straight back by your ears to prepare.

5. EXHALE and bring your arms toward your legs, and roll your back off the mat, reaching your hands to your feet and chest toward your thighs. Hold this "V" position for one second.

6. Slowly descend your back down toward the mat, while continually reaching your hands for your toes and "teasing" your back to the mat.

7. When your back is finally on the mat, reach your arms back overhead, and take a full INHALE. Sit up again, without a long rest in between.

8. Repeat 3 times.

LEG MODIFICATION:

With both knees together, bend one knee and place the foot on the floor and keep the other leg straight.

BREATH

Inhale: To prepare

Exhale: As you come up.

Inhale: At the top of your Teaser

Exhale: As you go down.

HELPFUL HINTS

⑥ Go for abdominal control instead of hip flexion. Think of hollowing out your abdomen, *like ice cream being scooped.*

⑥ Keep your shoulders down and gaze forward, toward the horizon, when seated in the "V" position.

⑥ Maintain Pilates stance to engage your inner and back thighs. Gently pull your tail under to roll back.

⑥ Teaser will also activate the hip flexor muscles, in front of the thighs. Bend your knees slightly to release some tension.

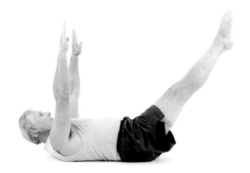
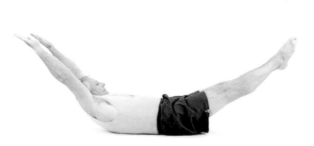

VISUALIZATION

Imagine a big heavy bowling ball resting in your lower belly. Balance it there, and use its weight to sink your lower back down while you simultaneously go up and over it.

CAUTION

- ☙ Ideally, your legs should be straight for this exercise; however, if you are new to the Teaser, there is nothing wrong with bending your knees.

- ☙ If you need to protect your lower back, definitely bend your knees.

- ☙ Only curl yourself halfway up and hold this position, then uncurl slowly down.

CHALLENGE

- ☙ Balance and hold the Teaser position while your core is sinking.

- ☙ Move through the exercise very slowly or with no momentum at all, and go down slower than you come up.

- ☙ Articulate your spine, feeling every bony protuberance of your vertebra while you descend.

- ☙ Change your breathing pattern: inhaling on the way up and exhaling on the way down.

SEATED CONSIDERATIONS

The Teaser directly targets the transversus, lower abdominal, muscle-the core of the powerhouse. This muscle is vital for abdominal support for the back, as well as pelvic stability and trunk strength.

TRANSITION TO NEXT EXERCISE

Turn over onto your stomach, keeping your legs long and arms reaching overhead. Place your forehead down.

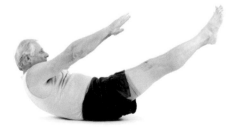
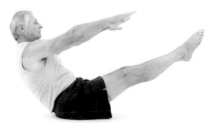

SWIMMING

Swimming strengthens the muscles besides the spine as well as the lower back.

THE EXERCISE

1. Lengthen your body long, especially from the waistband. Your arms and legs should be reaching in opposition, from your middle finger to your big toe!

2. Lift your right and left arms simultaneously. Hold for two counts.

3. Switch to the opposite arm and leg. Hold for two counts.

4. As you transition legs and arms, do not let them touch the mat. Keep the legs long.

5. Now, lift your head, as if you are taking it out of water. Keep the neck long. Then, start "swimming" by lifting your opposite arms and legs off the mat.

6. Flutter your arms and legs with length in the extremities and waist. As you swim, INHALE to a count of five, and EXHALE to a count of five. Keep the navel gently lifted and try not to rock.

7. Repeat.

8. Inhale and exhale for two more breathing cycles.

9. Rest: Sit back on your heels stretching the lower back. Be mindful that you are not letting your belly hang on your thighs.

VISUALIZATION

Imagine you are "swimming" with a fluttering kick.

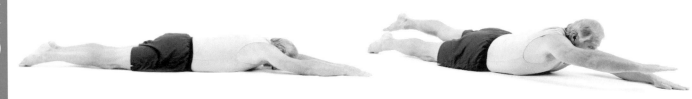

CAUTION/MODIFICAITONS

- ۞ Do not hyperextend your neck.

- ۞ If your back and/or neck get tired or sore: rest your forehead on your hands, with your elbows wide in a diamond shape. Only lift your chest and elbows up and down for a count of three. Repeat 3 times.

- ۞ For lower back or shoulder injury, limit your range of movement, and attempt the exercise cautiously or not at all.

- ۞ Just work the arms OR legs only; lifting one at a time.

CHALLENGE

- ۞ Lift higher in your chest and legs, while maintaining an abdominal contraction.

SEATED CONSIDERATIONS

Swimming will strengthen the lower back, thereby preventing back pain and help to avert the shoulders from rounding forward (like a Dowager's hump).

TRANSITION TO NEXT EXERCISE

Sit back on your bottom and heels to stretch the back round (rest pose). Then, sit on your bottom with your legs bent to the left to prepare for Mermaid.

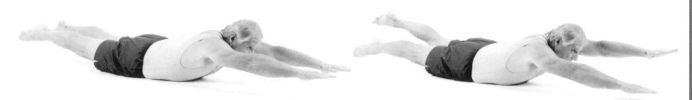

MERMAID

Mermaid will stretch the sides of your body and waist as well as open the hips and upper body in opposite directions.

THE EXERCISE

1. Sitting with your legs bent to the left side of your hips, hold your top ankle with your left hand. Stay square with both hips down. Look forward to keep the neck long and aligned with the spine.

2. Reach your right arm up against your head by your ear. INHALE and stretch your extended arm up and over to the left, lengthening from the waist. Stay lifted in your ribs and waist as you reach over.

3. EXHALE and return to an upright position and repeat 3 times, stretching deeper with each repetition.

4. Counter stretch by placing your right hand on the floor and lifting the left arm and waist over to the right.

5. Change sides and repeat 3 times on the opposite side.

VISUALIZATION

Imagine the arc of a rainbow, going up and overhead.

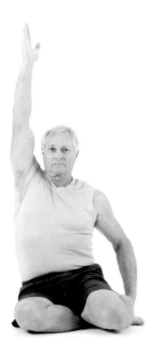 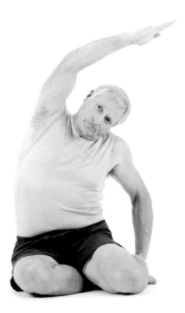

CAUTION

- ☙ Limit your range of movement if you feel extreme tightness.

- ☙ Be cautious with this exercise if you have knee joint problems. It may need to be omitted or do not tuck the shins in too tightly.

CHALLENGE

- ☙ After stretching up and over to one side, bend your extended elbow so that it touches your ear. Keep your ribs in as you reach over.

- ☙ Stacking the knees, one on top of the other, is ideal.

SEATED CONSIDERATIONS

After leaning over a desk all day, the oblique muscles get quite strained. The Mermaid is an excellent exercise for stretching and releasing the tension built up in this and other areas vulnerable to seated injury: the shoulders, the triceps muscle, and the upper back.

TRANSITION TO NEXT EXERCISE

Sit on your bottom at the front edge of your mat for The Seal.

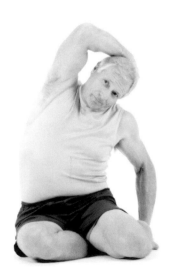
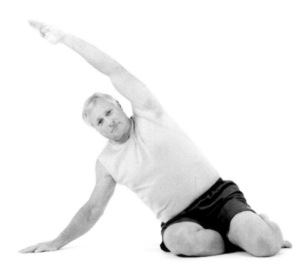

THE SEAL

The Seal massages the spine and internal organs, as well as tests your coordination and balance.

THE EXERCISE

1. Keep your feet together and open your knees apart in a diamond shape.
2. Place your hands in a prayer position, and dive them under your ankles, wrapping one hand around each ankle. Hold firmly.
3. Tilt back slightly, so your feet come off of the floor about two inches. Balance on the base of your sit bones and look at your feet.
4. Tuck your hips under so you are stretching your lower back. Look down into your belly and gently contract your abdominal muscles.
5. Clap your feet together three times.
6. INHALE and roll back to your shoulder blades. With your feet towards your head clap them together three times in this position. Do not roll onto the neck.
7. With the control you have from rolling on your spine, EXHALE and come back up to your sitting position.
8. Repeat for 5 rolls.

VARIATION

For an easier modification, you can simply clap the feet at the sitting position and not when you are back on your spine.

VISUALIZATION

Imagine your back rocking forward and backward like the base of a rocking chair.

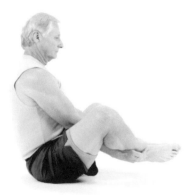
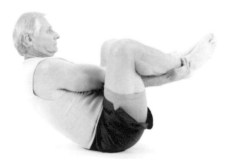

CAUTION

 ☙ Make sure you begin the exercise at the front end of your mat, so that when you roll back and forth you have extra mat behind you to protect your head, should it fall to the mat.

 ☙ As you roll back, your head should be in towards your chest.

 ☙ Don't throw your head back to roll onto your shoulder blades. Initiate the rolling from the abdominal muscles.

CHALLENGE

 ☙ Keep your stomach concave, especially as you come up to your seated position.

 ☙ Keep your shoulders down, especially as you roll up to your seated position.

 ☙ Work the hips by opening the legs, instead of just clapping the feet.

SEATED CONSIDERATIONS

The Seal will massage and stretch your back and hips and is an exceptional exercise that coincidentally stretches the wrists when your hands are wrapped around your ankles. (Pilates was a true genius, as he worked every body part!)

TRANSITION

After the last repetition, unwrap your hands, then cross your feet and arms, and roll up with one foot in front of the other. You will find yourself in the same standing position in which you began, with your arms in a "genie" stance.

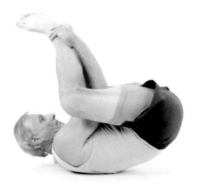 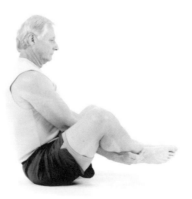

FINISHING YOUR WORKOUT

These exercises remind you to be aware of your posture, and focus on the importance of a long back and engaged abdominals. Doing so will promote a healthier, more vibrant you!

THE INVIGORATING COOL DOWN

THE EXERCISE

1. Stand tall, in the Pilates stance. Feel your ten toes evenly distributed on the floor.

2. Lengthen your neck, depress your shoulders, and lift your chest in a proud way.

3. Lengthen the sides of your waist. Keep the abdominal muscles engaged, lifting your navel in and up into your ribcage.

4. If you looked into a mirror laterally, you would want to see a plumb line straight from your ear, shoulder, hip and ankle all in perfect alignment.

5. Continue in this position and lean "into the wind," so that you come to the front of your toes.

6. Open your arms out to the side. Reach your middle fingers long to the opposite walls. Feel the opposition of your head to your heels and fingertip to fingertip.

7. Vigorously pump your arms forward with your <u>palms facing forward</u>. Repeat 10 times. Work dynamically; short and fast while maintaining a consistent breath.

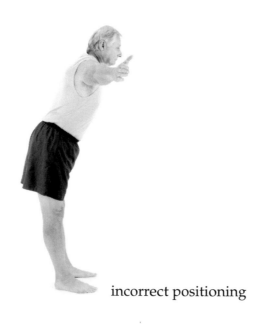 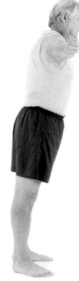

incorrect positioning   correct positioning

8. Change hand position and pump your arms, with your <u>palms facing backward</u>. Repeat 10 times.

9. Change your hand position so your <u>palms are facing up</u> to the ceiling, and pump energetically. Repeat 10 times.

10. Position your <u>palms down toward the floor</u> and pulse up and down forcefully. Repeat 10 times.

11. Finally, bring your arms down by your sides and roll your shoulders around forward for five circles and backward for five circles.

12. Take a full inhale and then a larger exhale.

13. Be on your way! Shoulders relaxed, chest proud, spine long, abdominals in and mind clear!

VISUALIZATION

Think of yourself as an arrow shooting through the sky, from the base of your heels to the top of your head.

palms facing forward

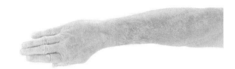

palms facing backward

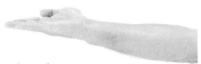

palms facing up

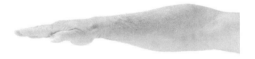

palms facing down

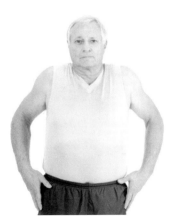 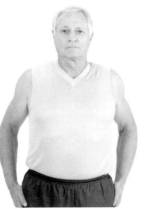

shoulder circles

THE WALL

A GREAT tension relieving and body aligning stretch…Do it any time of day!

THE EXERCISE

1. Stand with your back against a wall (approximately one foot step away) and place your feet in Pilates stance. Stand far enough away so that the entire length of your spine is flat against the wall.

2. Inhale and begin rolling your spine off the wall, one vertebra at a time, as if there was a piece of Velcro on the wall and you are peeling your spine off from it.

3. Roll down until you're your tail is the last part of your spine on the wall.

4. Allow the weight of your arms to hang to knee level. Imagine each hand is holding a light bowling ball. Circle the arms freely in a small circle five times. Switch directions for five more circles. Release your head and neck.

5. Roll your spine back up the wall, imagining you are placing it onto the Velcro with slight pressure. Feel the back of your head against the wall.

6. Walk your feet back to the wall and stand tall.

7. Lift through your long spine, lengthen your neck, open your shoulders and expand your chest. Breath. And walk away proud and pleased!

HELPFUL HINTS

Pull your navel in and up and maintain this connection throughout the entire exercise.

⑥ Breath effortlessly throughout the entire exercise, especially when your head is down.

⑥ Bend your knees slightly to ease any tension.

⑥ 1 or 2 pound weights can be used in each hand for more challenge and stretch.

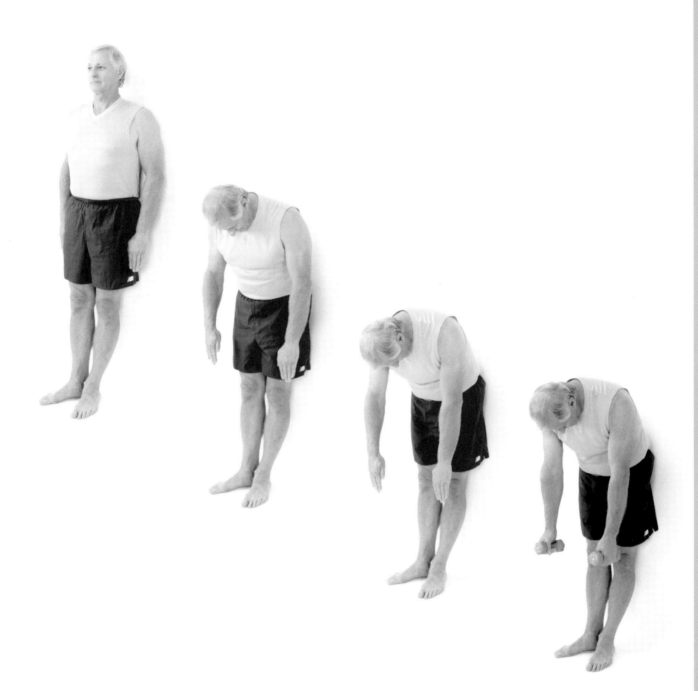

THE MID-DAY MINDFUL WORKOUT

Don't underestimate the power of these simple stretches that can be done throughout the day, whenever you have a free hand or an extra few minutes. As you integrate Pilates into your life, commit to building these stretches into your schedule. You'll not only enhance the value of your regular workouts, you'll increase the effectiveness of your work.

HELPFUL HINTS

- Never force a stretch; relax as much as possible using the breath to facilitate the stretch. Exhale on the effort.
- Breath naturally, but be mindful of keeping it slow and deep.
- Let the stretch occur naturally; that is, get a slight stretch first, then enhance the stretch once you feel the muscle relax.
- Hold most stretches for about 3 breathing cycles or about 5-10 seconds each stretch.
- Be kind to your body as we are not the same everyday; some days we may be tighter than another.
- Stretch routinely, especially on a daily basis.
- Perform each exercise on both sides of the body.

HAND STRETCHES

(To help prevent Carpal Tunnel Syndrome)

WRIST FLEXOR AND EXTENSOR STRETCH

This exercise will relieve hand and wrist strain.

THE EXERCISE

1. Straighten your elbow and pull your fingers backward as far as possible, with your opposite hand supporting your palm.

2. Hold for about 8 seconds and repeat 2 times

VARIATION

> To counter the stretch, place your palm on the outside of your opposite hand and press down, gently bringing your palm closer to the inside wrist.

HELPFUL HINT

Keep your fingers straight. Work from your wrist, and not just your fingers.

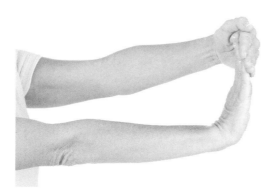
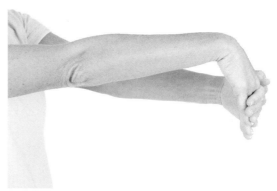

THUMB STRETCH

This exercise, and the next, opens and lengthens the tissues that are most often shortened by doing repetitive tasks.

THE EXERCISE

1. Gently pull your thumb away from the index finger, allowing the web between the two to stretch.
2. Hold for about 8 seconds and repeat 2 times.

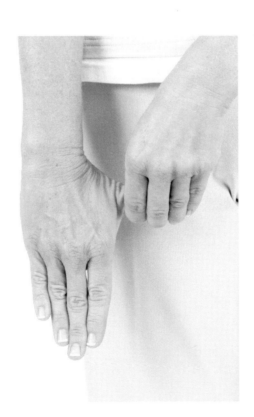

INDIVIDUAL FINGER FLEXOR AND EXTENSOR STRETCH

THE EXERCISE

1. Flex each individual finger, shortening the distance between the finger and the palm, with the opposite thumb and/or fingers. Release and repeat gaining more stretch with each repetition. Perform one to two sets with the palm up, sideways, or with the palm down.

2. Extend each finger backward toward the back of the hand. Stretch one finger at a time. You will notice that each digit will stretch to different lengths. This exercise is most productive with the palm facing down.

3. Hold each finger about 5 seconds and repeat and release for one to two sets.

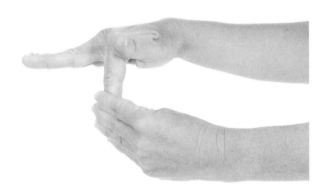

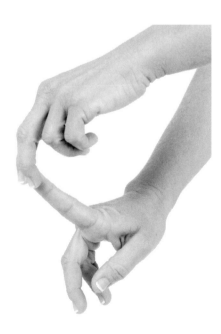

FISTED WRIST STRETCH

This stretch is excellent for countering the constant tension on the wrist.

THE EXERCISE

1. Extend your arm in front and make a fist with one hand. With the opposite hand gently press on the outside of the hand, drawing the hand down. Flex the wrist as much as comfortably possible.

2. Repeat 4 times, feeling the stretch go further with each repetition.

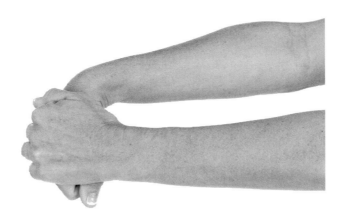

OPEN HAND STRETCH/OPEN HAND STRETCH

This exercise brings circulation and vitality to the hands.

THE EXERCISE

1. Spread your fingers as wide apart as physically possible. Hold for two to three seconds. Release. Make a tight fist and begin again.

2. Hold for about two to three seconds and release.

3. Repeat 5 times.

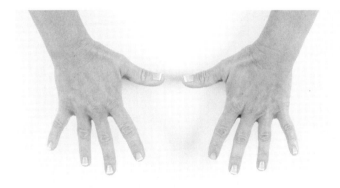

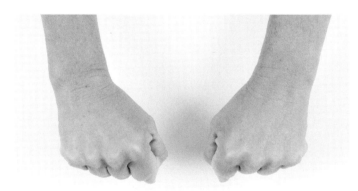

NECK STRETCHES

Stretching the neck improves range of movement and motion, a vital necessity for these most often overworked muscles of the seated professional. Stretching the neck will ease stiffness, reduce stress and provide relief for cervical muscle tension.

EAR TO SHOULDER

THE EXERCISE

1. Bring your ear directly over to your shoulder.
2. Keep your eyes directed forward to prevent rotation of the head.
3. Repeat four times, holding about 5 seconds for each repetition.

> **HELPFUL HINTS**
>
> ◎ These wonderful stretches can be performed any time of day.
> ◎ Take time to feel the stretch; don't rush it.

BREATH

Exhale: On the furthest part of the stretch and hold for about 5 seconds.

VARIATION

For further stretch: place the opposite hand on the side of the head and gently assist in the pull.

For even further stretch: pull the opposite shoulder down towards the floor. Inhale while returning to the neutral position.

VISUALIZATION

Imagine your head arching over like a rainbow. Keep it in the frontal plane at all times, and maintain your abdominals slightly engaged to support the stretch.

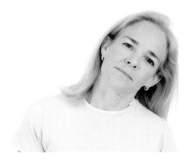

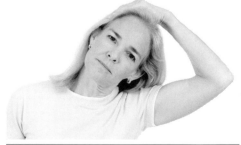

VARIATION

CHIN TO ARMPIT

THE EXERCISE

1. Turn your head slightly to one side and bring your chin to your armpit.
2. Repeat 4 times, holding about 5 seconds for each repetition.
3. Assist with the other hand, after a few repetitions, to lengthen the neck muscles further.

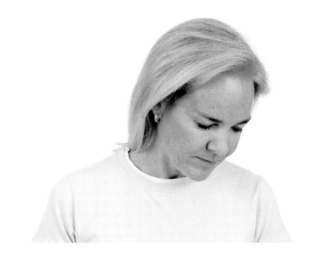

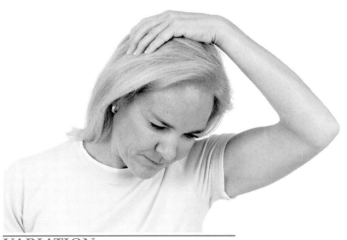

VARIATION

EAR TO CHEST

THE EXERCISE

1. Turn your head slightly to one side.
2. Bring your ear towards your chest (nipple).
3. Repeat 4 times, holding about 5 seconds for each repetition.

VARIATION

To stretch further: place your hand on the side of your head and gently pull. Return to starting position and repeat.

BREATH

Exhale: On the stretch.

HELPFUL HINTS

⑥ Do not lift your shoulder or twist your trunk while performing the exercise; keep the abdominal muscles gently contracted.

⑥ Holding the underside of a stool or chair and gently pulling with the opposite hand will lower the shoulder and facilitate the stretch.

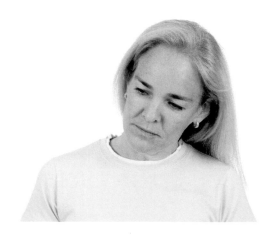
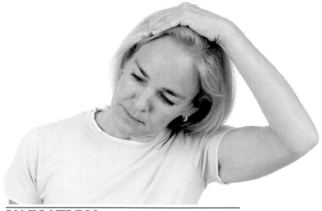

VARIATION

NECK FLEXION

THE EXERCISE

1. Bring your chin directly to your chest, and draw the chin down, while stretching the back of your neck.
2. Contribute to the stretch by placing the hand on the back of the head.
3. Release and return too neutral.
4. Repeat 4 times, holding about 5 seconds for each repetition.

VARIATION

Enhance the stretch by being mindful of the downward draw of the shoulder blades along the upper back.

CAUTION

This stretch is to be limited if the person is frequently looking down, such as reading or looking at a keyboard. Stretching the muscles, however, can be helpful in relieving tightness.

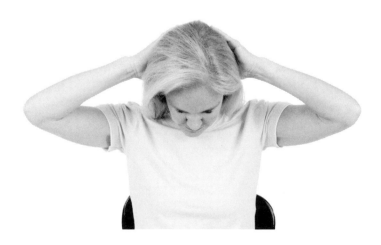

HEAD SEMI-CIRCLES

For relieving tight muscles around the upper part of the neck.

THE EXERCISE

1. Beginning with your chin down, draw your nose up towards the right shoulder and then towards the ceiling.

2. Repeat to the other side for four complete cycles.

VISUALIZATION

Make the shape of a horseshoe.

CAUTION

Do not compress the neck vertebra by putting your head all the way backward. This places unnecessary stress on the tendons, ligaments and bones of the neck.

HELPFUL HINT

Keep the abdominals contracted to prevent the entire spine from stretching forward. This stretch is specific for the cervical vertebra.

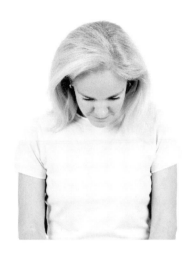
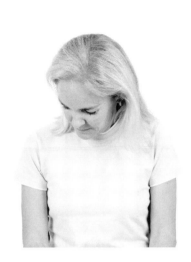
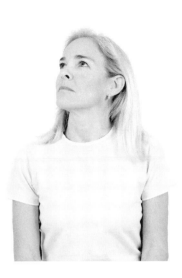
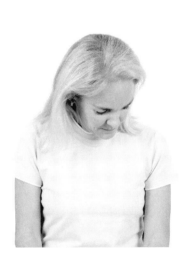
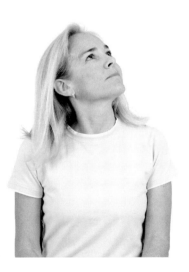

SHOULDER STRETCHES

Keeping the shoulders loose and relaxed will help you feel less stressed and tense.

SHOULDER SHRUGS

THE EXERCISE

1. Lift and lower the shoulders up and down.
2. Repeat 5 times inhaling on the lift, holding for 3 seconds and exhaling on the lowering.

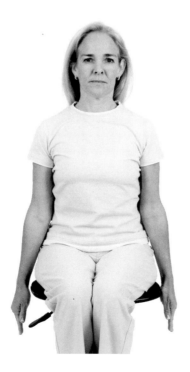
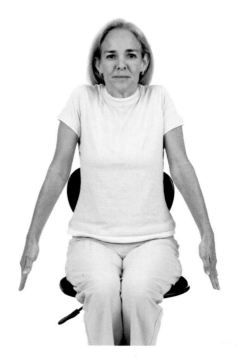

ARM ACROSS CHEST

(Straight-arm or 90° elbow bend)

THE EXERCISE

1. Bring your arm straight up to a horizontal position, across your chest.
2. Use the opposite hand and arm to gently pull the arm across to the opposite shoulder.
3. Repeat three times and hold for two breath counts in each of these positions.

VARIATION

Rotating the thumb downward and lowering the arm toward the breastbone will further enhance the stretch.

HELPFUL HINT

Keep both shoulder blades down and back throughout the exercise, and do not turn the body.

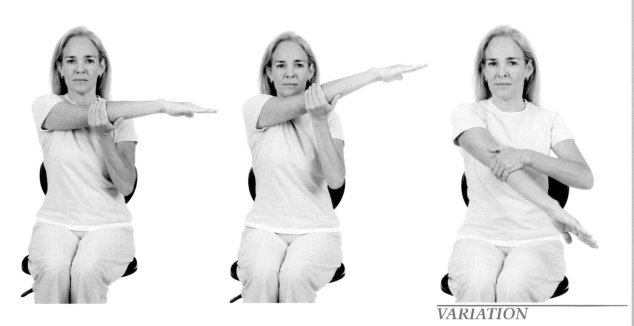

VARIATION

SHOULDER AND CHEST STRETCH

To stretch your arms and chest muscles.

THE EXERCISE

1. Interlace your fingers behind your back and hold your palms facing each other. Inhale as you lift and press your arms up. Hold two seconds, and exhale on the release.

2. Repeat four cycles .

HELPFUL HINTS

⑥ The breathing pattern can be reversed. Either way, Remember to breathe!

⑥ Keep the hand apart & lift, if it is too difficult to clasp your hands together.

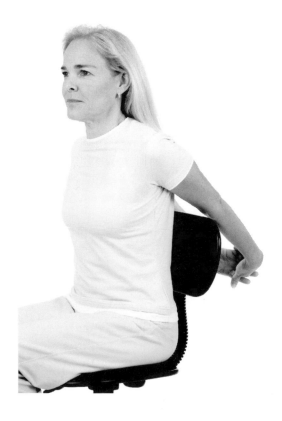

ONE ARM UP AND ONE ARM DOWN

THE EXERCISE

1. Stretch one arm up to the ceiling and the other arm down towards the floor. Reach both arms away from one another.

2. Hold for three counts and switch to the other side, hold for three counts. Repeat each cycle 5 times.

HELPFUL HINT

Think of a tug-of-war between the opposing fingers, arms and side body.

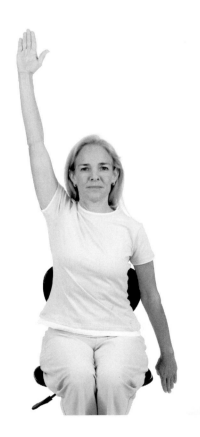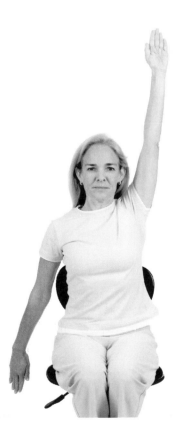

CHEST EXPANSION

This exercise improves breath and invigorates your upper body.

THE EXERCISE

1. Sit very tall in your chair. Pull the shoulder blades gently down and back along the back ribs. Place your hands by your sides, palms facing backward.

2. FULLY Inhale and press your arms back and lift them up to the ceiling. Hold the breath about 2 seconds and slowly release the arms down, controlling the downward movement with mindfulness.

3. Repeat 5 times, inhaling on the lift and exhaling on the lower. Hold the breath in between.

HELPFUL HINT

Work both positively as well as negatively.

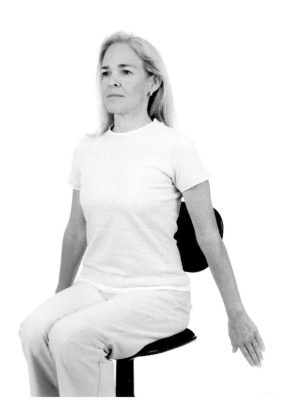

SHAVING

This exercise works the upper back and arm muscles. If you are already tight in your upper back, this exercise may be omitted.

THE EXERCISE

1. Bring the index finger and thumbs together to create a triangular shape with your hands. Keep this connection.

2. Bring the held hands up to the ceiling. Then bring the clasped fingers to the nape of the neck or the crown of the head.

3. Straighten and bend the elbows widely, working the upper back and arms.

4. Repeat 5 times, inhaling on the lift while straightening the arms and exhaling on the lowering, allowing the elbows to open.

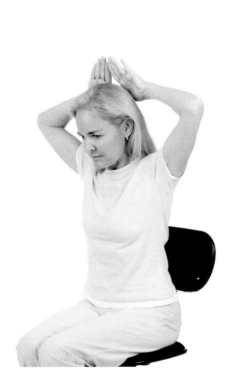 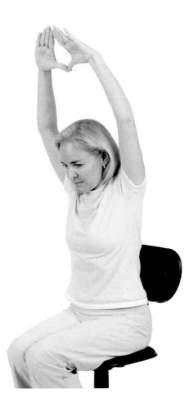

TRICEPS STRETCH

Specifically stretches the upper back of the arm.

THE EXERCISE

1. Bend your elbow and place your hand on your shoulder.
2. Lift your elbow up to the ceiling, allowing your opposite hand to facilitate the lift and stretch.
3. Hold at the top for about two seconds.
4. Release and repeat eight times.

VARIATION

Keep the bent elbow lifting to the ceiling. With the opposite hand providing support, straighten and bend the elbow, lifting and lowering the forearm. Hold the bent arm for about two seconds, exhaling on the stretch. Release and repeat about eight times. Repeat for the opposite arm.

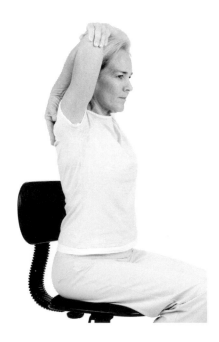

SHOULDER CIRCLES

This exercise can be done any time, anywhere as a great stress release of your body and mind.

THE EXERCISE

1. Sitting erect, take a full inhale and slowly exhale.
2. Lift your shoulders up, back, forward and around to make a complete circle.
3. Return to the starting position.
4. Change directions.
5. Repeat five times in each direction.

BREATH

Inhale: Raise and roll your shoulders back.

Exhale: Upon completion of the circle.

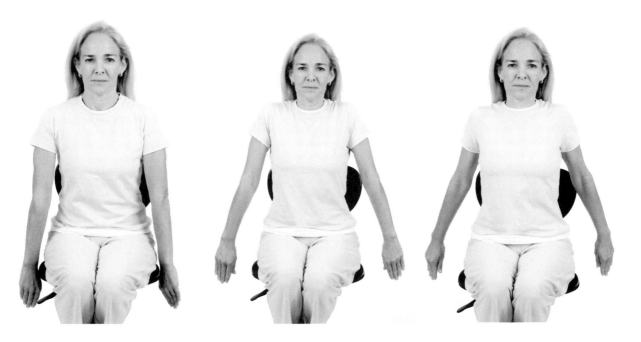

UPPER BODY STRETCHES

FINGERS CLASPED AND ARMS UP TO THE CEILING

THE EXERCISE

1. Clasp your fingers in front of you and turn your palms outward.
2. Lift your arms straight up to the ceiling.
3. Hold for about two seconds.
4. Lower your arms down.
5. Repeat five times.

BREATH

Inhale: Lift the arms.

Exhale: Lower the arms.

HELPFUL HINT

This is a great "anytime" stretch!

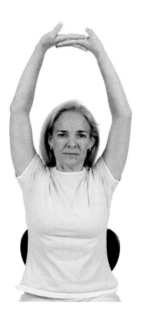

LATERAL TRUNK STRETCH

THE EXERCISE

1. Clasp your left hand around your right wrist and lift your arms up overhead.
2. Sitting tall with your abdominals slightly contracted, bend your torso laterally to the right side.
3. Repeat four times.
4. Stretch the opposite side, switching hands.
5. Repeat four times.

VARIATION

1. Perform exercise as above, while in the standing position.
2. The exercise can be performed with arms down or one arm overhead. Both arms overhead is the most challenging of the stretches.
3. Perform the exercise with opposite wrist holding for a deeper stretch.

BREATH

Inhale: On the lift.

Exhale: On the lateral stretch. Hold for about two seconds.

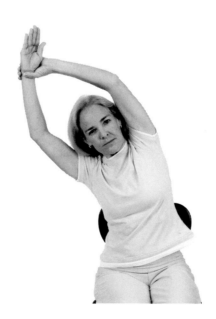

UPPER TRUNK EXTENSION

THE EXERCISE

Sitting:

1. Hold your hands behind your head and sit tall.
2. Slowly inhale and lift your spine up and slightly backward to a point of maximal stretch.
3. Hold for about three seconds.
4. Come back to your original position and repeat five times.

Standing:

1. Place your hands on the back of your hips and gently lift and extend your back up and backward.
2. Hold about three seconds and return to your original position.
3. Repeat five times.

BREATH

Inhale: On the lift.

Exhale: On the return.

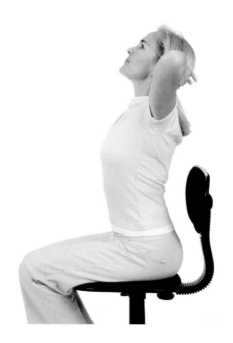

LATERAL ROTATION

THE EXERCISE

Sitting:

1. Sitting tall, open your knees, and rotate your spine to one side, lifting as you twist.
2. For added stretch, place your hands under the chair seat, between the knees and backrest, to pull further. (*Variation #1*)
3. Keep your bottom stable, in the center of the chair, by firmly pressing your lower torso against the back of the chair.
4. Repeat to the other side after five repetitions.

VARIATION

1. Place your arms in a "T" position to facilitate the reach and stretch.
2. For a further seated twist: Cross one knee over the other and rotate laterally.

> **HELPFUL HINT**
>
> On all rotations, where you look, your body will follow. Be mindful of your eye direction.

BREATH

Inhale: On the twist. Hold for two seconds.

Exhale: On the release.

CAUTION

Keep your eyes looking to the horizon or middle of a wall. Do not look up or down, as that will unnecessarily twist the upper, cervical, spine.

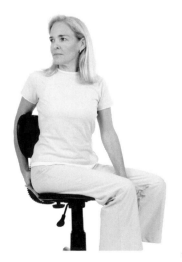
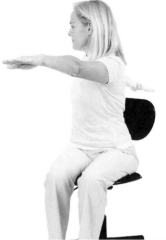
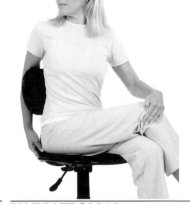

VARIATION #1   *VARIATION #2*

TRUNK FLEXION

This stretch is superb for the seated professional with lower back tightness; however, should be limited in repetitions if the upper spine and shoulders are already rolled forward.

THE EXERCISE

1. Sit on a chair seat and slowly lower your chest toward your thighs, hinging at the hips. Your hands may remain on your knees or along the side of them.
2. Bring your head between your arms and toward your knees. Hold 2 counts and stretch.
3. Inhale to your original position.
4. Repeat five times.

VARIATION

Let the arms fall between the legs to add natural weight to the stretch.

CAUTION

Exercise care to the spine if it is inflexible.

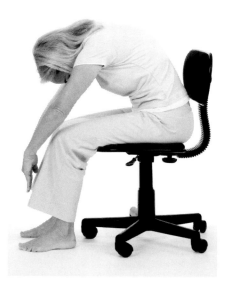
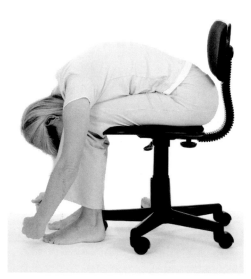

ABDOMINAL CONTRACTIONS

THE EXERCISE

1. Pull your navel toward your spine and sit tall, with your shoulders relaxed and drawn down.

2. Repeat five to ten times, holding the contraction for 3-5 seconds each.

BREATH

Exhale: On the contraction, bringing your naval to your spine, narrowing your waistband.

HELPFUL HINT

This exercise can be done throughout the day.

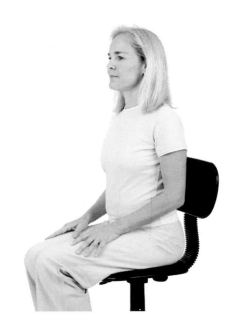 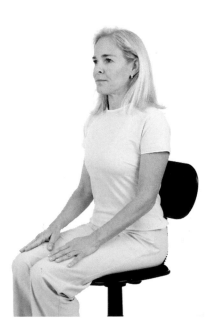

MY HOPE FOR YOU

As you begin to integrate the stretches and exercises in this book with your own body knowledge and lifestyle, you are beginning a new chapter in your own spinal story. Take note. Ask questions. Mostly, be mindful.

I wish you a career filled with health, balance, and most of all, personal success. When you walk into work each day with your head held high, posture upright and your mind filled with good intentions, I hope you feel a renewed sense of vitality and happiness. Breathe deeply and keep moving—good health will be your greatest reward.